D0473806

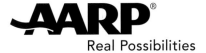

Real Possibilities

Memory
Activity
Book

**Engaging ways to stimulate the brain,
for people living with memory loss or dementia**

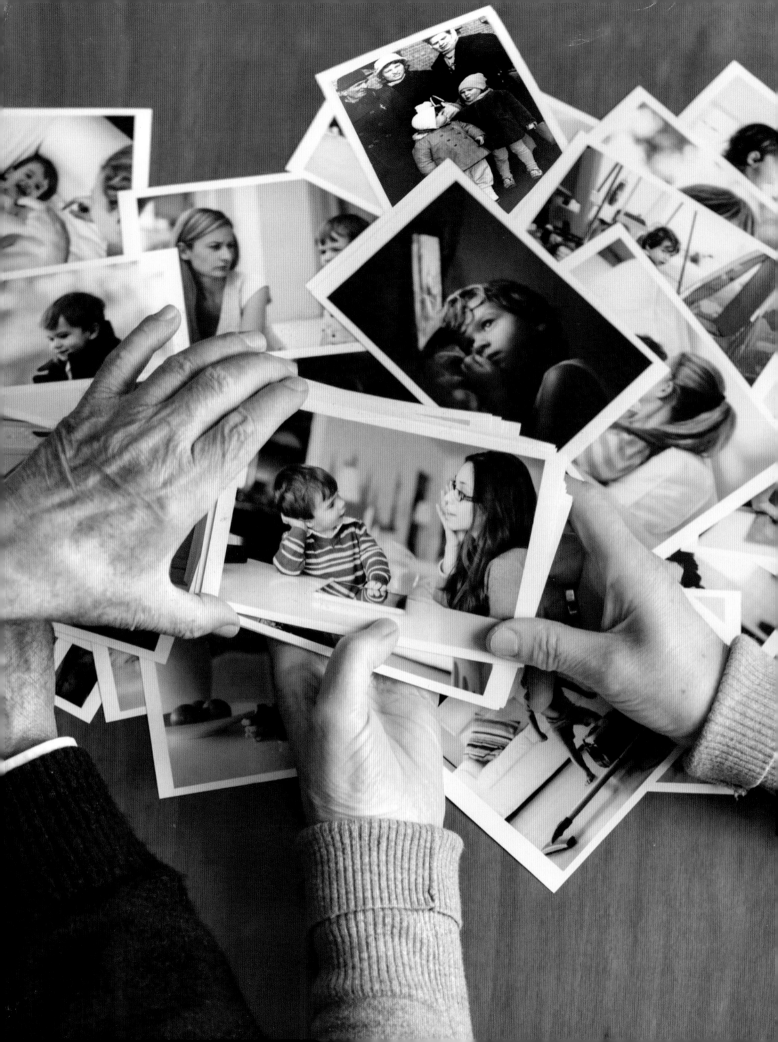

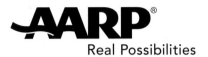

AARP®
Real Possibilities

Memory
Activity
Book

Engaging ways to stimulate the brain, for people living with memory loss or dementia

Helen Lambert

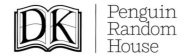

Penguin Random House

DK UK

Project art editor Francis Wong
Project editors Annelise Evans, Miezan van Zyl
US editor Karyn Gerhard
Senior designer Sharon Spencer
Senior editor Helen Fewster
Proofreader Ruth O'Rourke Jones
Jacket design development manager
Sophia MTT
Jacket editor Claire Gell
Producer, pre-production Andy Hilliard
Senior producer Alex Bell
Managing editor Angeles Gavira Guerrero
Managing art editor Michael Duffy
Associate publishing director Liz Wheeler
Art director Karen Self
Design director Phil Ormerod
Publishing director Jonathan Metcalf

For Nana
Author Helen Lambert
Cofio Dementia Training

DK INDIA

Senior designers Mahua Mandal,
Vaibhav Rastogi
Editors Arpita Dasgupta, Priyanjali Narain
Assistant art editors Rabia Ahmad,
Simar Dhamija
Jacket designer Tanya Mehrotra
Jackets editorial coordinator
Priyanka Sharma
Managing jackets editor Saloni Singh
DTP designer Ashok Kumar
Senior DTP designer Harish Aggarwal,
Vishal Bhatia
Assistant Picture Researcher
Vishal Ghavri
Managing Picture Researcher
Taiyaba Khatoon
Senior managing editor Rohan Sinha
Managing art editor Sudakshina Basu
Pre-production manager Balwant Singh
Production manager Pankaj Sharma

First American Edition, 2018
Published in the United States by DK Publishing
345 Hudson Street, New York, New York 10014

Copyright © 2018 Dorling Kindersley Limited
DK, a Division of Penguin Random House LLC
18 19 20 21 22 10 9 8 7 6 5 4 3 2 1
001 – 305946 – Nov/2018

A catalog record for this book
is available from the Library of Congress.
ISBN: 978-1-4654-6922-9

DK books are available at special discounts
when purchased in bulk for sales
promotions, premiums, fund-raising, or
educational use. For details, contact:
DK Publishing Special Markets, 345 Hudson
Street, New York, New York 10014
SpecialSales@dk.com

Printed and bound in China

A WORLD OF IDEAS:
SEE ALL THERE IS TO KNOW

www.dk.com

PLEASE NOTE

This book is intended for informational purposes only and is not intended to be a substitute for professional or medical advice. The suggestions for activities in this book are based on research by the publisher, but the publisher is not engaged in rendering personal advice to individual readers in relation to medical or other matters. Each reader should be aware that the ability to undertake activities (or the extent to which activities can be undertaken) diminishes over time for people living with dementia, and abilities and activities should therefore be reassessed from time to time. Readers should always take the range of their abilities into account before adopting any suggestion in this book. Before undertaking any exercise, readers are advised to seek the advice of their doctor. The publisher and AARP cannot accept, expressly disclaim, and deny any liability for any loss, injury, or damage that is sustained by readers in consequence of adopting any suggestions or of using the information in this book.

Contents

Preface

You'll find a lot of conflicting information about brain health out there. Scientists haven't found a miracle cure to keep our brains sharp. But one thing we do know is that keeping engaged and connected can help. That's where "The Memory Activity Book" comes in.

Here you'll find a collection of more than 70 engaging and fun projects, designed to boost brain health for people living with memory loss, Alzheimer's disease, or another form of dementia, and for their relatives, friends, and caregivers. While activities of this nature have not been proven to stop dementia or memory loss, they may slow the progression or improve the symptoms. Equally important, they provide meaningful ways to spend time with loved ones. The benefits of trying these activities are numerous.

■ Completing the activities with family members, loved ones, or caregivers fosters a sense of connection and togetherness that is important for emotional well-being.
■ The activities let you enjoy life in the moment, while it is happening.
■ The more physical activities support overall health, which in turn can improve brain health.
■ Crafting activities help you practice skills and make things that will help you function better in everyday life, now and in the future.

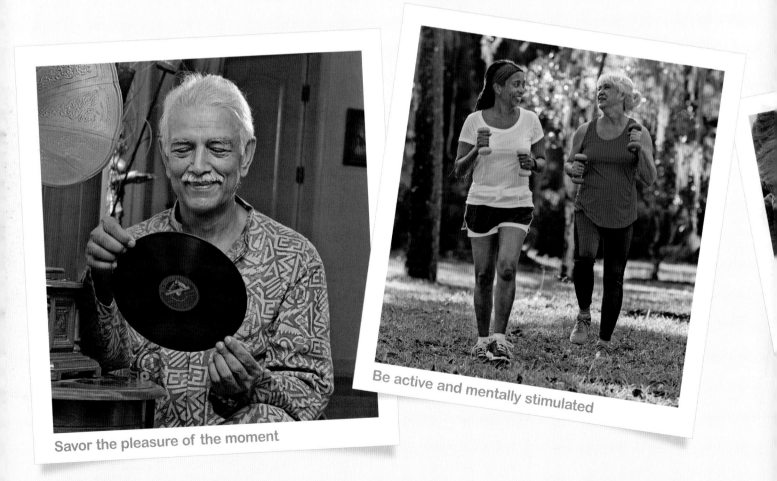

Savor the pleasure of the moment

Be active and mentally stimulated

The activities each offer at-a-glance guidance: how long they take, whether they're to do alone or with others, the skill level, what you'll need to do them, and how they help. They are grouped according to themes:

■ Out and About: These activities are more physical in nature and can help support mental well-being and improve mood by increasing blood flow to your brain.

■ Revisiting the Past: Reminiscing helps trigger memories and emotions, and these activities let you connect with loved ones and enjoy exploring personal and family history together.

■ Music and Dance: Use the power of music to bring you joy, connect with others, and express yourself.

■ Puzzles and Games: These activities stimulate your brain and may boost your ability to think, reason, concentrate, and deal with tasks.

■ Arts and Crafts: Feel the satisfaction of working with your hands and producing something beautiful and useful while stimulating your senses.

Flip though the book and find an activity that interests you and fits your abilities. Then jump right in and get started!

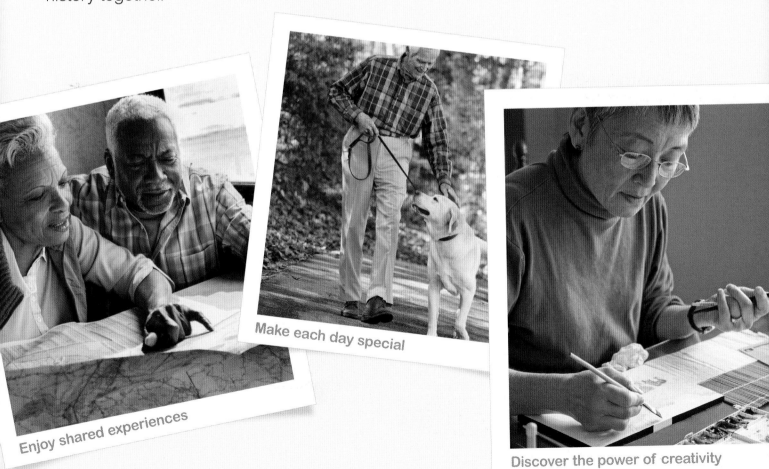

Enjoy shared experiences

Make each day special

Discover the power of creativity

INTRODUCTION

How memories work

The human memory is complex and not fully understood. To remember something, the entire brain engages in a series of specific tasks so that we can recall events that have shaped the person we are.

Short-term memory

We have many types of memories that do different things. Our immediate memory is unconscious and takes in information from the senses—sight, sound, touch, smell, and taste—in seconds. It then consolidates relevant information into short-term memory.

The short-term, or working, memory holds on to information for 30–60 seconds. This is long enough to add up a sum in your head or write down a telephone number. It is also believed to sift out details that we don't need to remember. However, short-term memory can hold on to only five to eight pieces of information at a time, so if you are distracted, you easily forget that information.

Long-term memory

In the cerebral cortex, a long-term memory is encoded and stored by forging connections between brain cells. These connections and the memory are stronger if we rehearse the information or if it involves emotion.

Storing memories
One theory of how memory works is that short-term memory takes data from the immediate memory, organizes it, and makes it a long-term memory that can be retrieved at a later point.

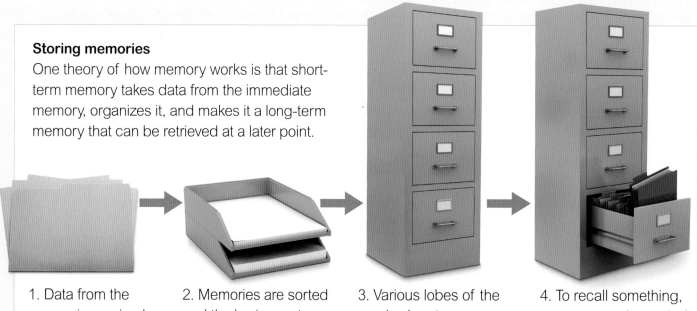

1. Data from the senses is received by the brain, which organizes it to make short-term memories.

2. Memories are sorted and the brain creates a chain of electrical and chemical connections between brain cells.

3. Various lobes of the cerebral cortex, or gray matter, in the brain store many different types of encoded memories.

4. To recall something, your unconscious mind searches for and retrieves the relevant encoded memory.

Types of long-term memories

We have several types of long-term memories to remember different kinds of events, information, or feelings.

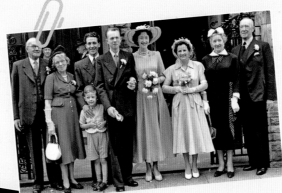

Episodic memory

We use our memory of events or episodes in our lives to remember our wedding day, the birth of a child, a schoolteacher, or that we had eggs for breakfast.

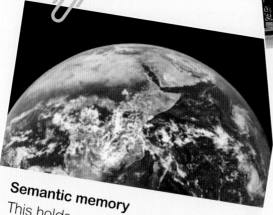

Semantic memory

This holds our general knowledge, information that we have learned over the years, and the things we just know to be true. For example, it tells us that the world is round.

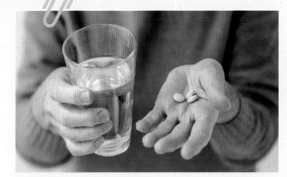

Prospective memory

Prospective memory allows us to remember to do something in the future, such as to go to an appointment or to take medication.

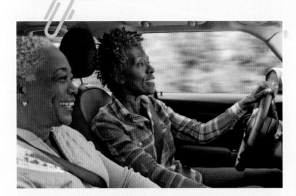

Procedural memory

This allows us to carry out learned tasks, such as driving a car or making a cup of coffee. We don't think about many things we do each day; we just know how to do them.

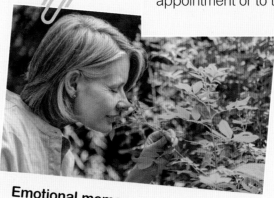

Emotional memory

Emotional memory, of positive or negative feelings, may be triggered when we see, hear, touch, smell, or taste something that reminds us of a particular time in our life.

What is dementia?

Dementia is an umbrella term used to describe the symptoms caused by different diseases and conditions that affect brain function. In all types of dementia, the brain is gradually damaged and symptoms worsen over time.

Symptoms of dementia

The symptoms of dementia vary from person to person, and it is impossible to predict what impact dementia will have on your life. In the early stage, changes are subtle. You may notice your memory is less reliable and just chalk it up to age, but it may become more significant over time. Other symptoms include:

■ Having difficulty managing money or balancing the checkbook.

■ Becoming lost in once-familiar places or struggling to recognize acquaintances.

■ Forgetting where you put things.

■ Repeating yourself often.

■ Changes in your vision.

■ Communication difficulties.

■ A change in cognitive skills, with everyday tasks becoming more challenging.

■ Becoming less steady on your feet.

■ Noticable changes in mood, such as feeling depressed or anxious, or behavior.

Common types of dementia

Alzheimer's disease and vascular dementia are most common, but there are probably more than a hundred different types.

■ **Alzheimer's disease** affects the entire brain over a period of years, with a gradual decline in function. The brain shrinks as brain cells die, affecting the hippocampus (site of short-term memory), so memory impairment is one of the first symptoms.

■ **Vascular dementia** is caused by a disruption to the brain's blood supply. Unlike Alzheimer's disease, vascular dementia causes only patchy brain damage, so some parts of the brain are not affected.

■ **Mixed dementia** involves Alzheimer's disease and another type of dementia, commonly vascular dementia.

■ **Dementia with Lewy bodies** combines some cognitive decline associated with Alzheimer's disease and symptoms that are similar to those of Parkinson's disease. These symptoms include difficulties with mobility, stiffness, and shaking. Hallucinations are also a common symptom.

■ **Frontotemporal dementia** results from damage to the front part of the brain initially, causing people to behave "out of character." They may not censor their thoughts and feelings as they used to, saying hurtful things, swearing, or behaving in a disinhibited way. Communication difficulties are common.

Parts of the brain affected

The brain is a highly complex and specialized organ. Damage to different parts of the brain impacts someone with dementia in various ways.

■ **The hippocampus** is crucial to receiving information from the short-term memory and laying down new long-term memories. It also helps us map where one thing is in relation to another and how we get from A to B.

■ **The frontal lobe** is the part of the brain that allows us to reason; make decisions; weigh risks; initiate sequence and complete tasks; control thoughts and reactions; and censor behavior.

■ **The parietal lobe** interprets information from the senses, enabling us to read, use numbers, and recognize pain.

■ **The temporal lobe** is involved in memory storage and language skills, hearing, and emotion.

■ **The occipital lobe** is mainly concerned with interpreting what the eye sees.

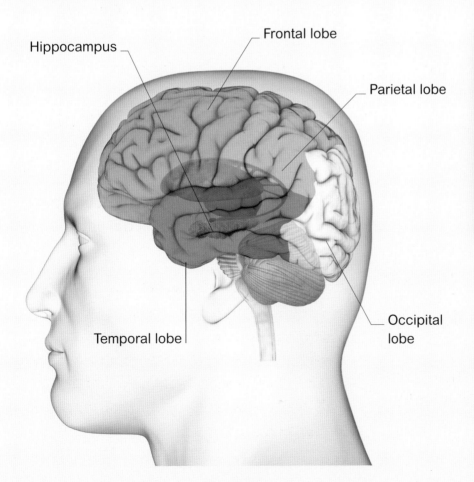

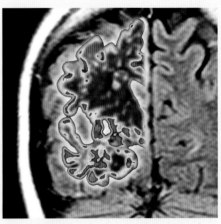

▲ A brain scan shows half the brain (in orange) of a person with Alzheimer's disease, overlaid on a healthy brain. It is clear how much the damaged brain has shrunk.

◄ Billions of brain cells control everything we think, feel, and do. Dementia symptoms vary based on where damage occurs.

Living with dementia

It may be possible to slow the progression of dementia and take steps to minimize the impact the condition has on your everyday life. Even so, symptoms fluctuate and there will be good and bad days.

Plan ahead

Focusing on meaningful activities you can do may help to maintain your quality of life and well-being. You may be able to slow cognitive and memory decline by physical exercise and by challenging your brain. Establishing routines may help maintain your independence. Prepare memory labels and signs (see pages 204–207) to remind you of the steps involved in tasks such as using the washing machine or to indicate the contents of a cupboard.

Use a calendar

▶ Plan ahead by using a calendar and place signs throughout your home to alleviate feeling disorientated.

Make memory signs

Assistive technology

A wide range of items, often technology-based, is available to help you stay independent. These include night/day clocks that indicate when it is time to get out of bed and alerts that allow you to call for help when in distress. Safe walking technologies with GPS devices help you find your way—or be found if you get lost or into difficulty: they can make the difference between staying at home and going for a walk.

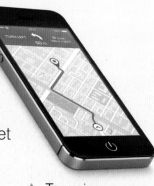

▲ Try using a GPS app on your phone.

Manage risk

As dementia progresses, some things will become more difficult to do. It is important to acknowledge changes and adapt certain activities to your changing abilities. Focus on what you can do, rather that what you cannot do. However, many things we do in life involve risk, so it should be your aim to minimize risk, rather than eliminating every activity that involves a slight risk. You may find that having someone with you helps you to feel more confident.

Maintain relationships

Social interaction supports brain health. Maintaining positive relationships also helps you avoid loneliness and isolation. It can also help you to retain a sense of self—your feelings about who you are as a person. Your role within any relationship does not have to change. Sharing activities with another person who can help you may give you confidence to try new things or to continue doing things that are important to you. Participating in social activities with family or friends, such as playing a game or going on an outing, also may help you maintain your communication skills.

USEFUL TIPS

Declutter your cupboards and work spaces to make it easier to find things

Make a list of daily, weekly, and monthly tasks. Check them off as you do them

▼ Maintaining relationships with family and friends is fundamentally important because social contact keeps you feeling connected to those around you.

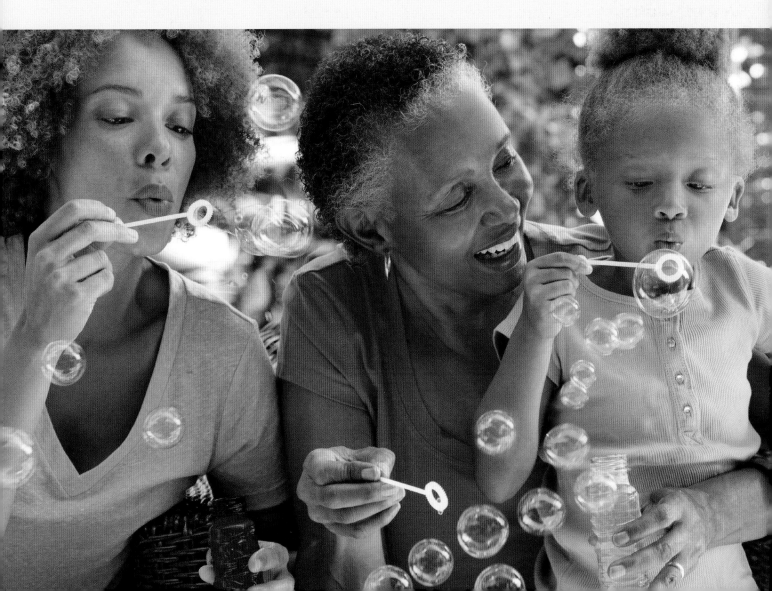

How activities help

As human beings, we have an innate need to be active and occupied. Activity of all kinds, from doing a craft project to making a cup of coffee, may benefit both our physical and mental well-being. Inactivity, or irregular activity, can lead to agitation or irritability.

Keeping fit and healthy

Try to be as physically active as you can. This could involve going for a run or swim, riding a bicycle, and playing a team sport, but also more gentle exercise, such as taking a walk in the garden or even just moving around more in the house. The benefits of exercise include:

▼ Biking increases blood flow to the brain and helps to maintain your gross-motor skills.

■ Maintaining mobility, strength, balance, and good posture.

■ Reducing aches and pains, and also reducing the risk of falls.

■ Support of heart health.

■ Increased flow of oxygenated blood to the brain, slowing down cognitive decline and memory loss.

■ Increased appetite, better digestion, and reducing risks of constipation.

■ Improved quality of sleep.

Staying socially active

Activities frequently provide you with opportunities to socialize with family and friends. This can boost your confidence and spirits, make you feel better about yourself, and stop you from becoming isolated and lonely. It is easier to establish a routine if you commit to regularly meeting with friends or family. Sharing activities and engaging with others may also help you keep your cognitive and communication skills sharper for longer.

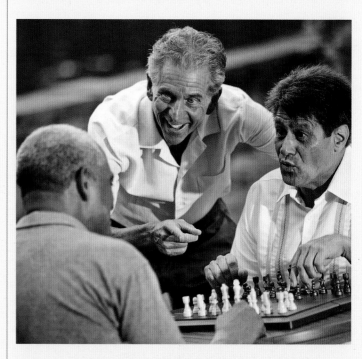

▲ Participating in social activities supports brain health, is fun, and allows you to maintain your communication and social skills.

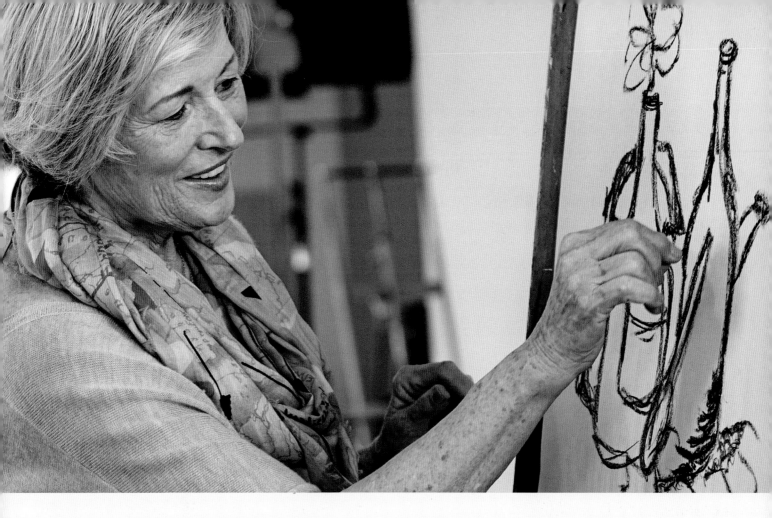

Improving cognitive skills

The brain uses cognitive skills to make sense of the world. You may be able to slow the decline of these skills by doing activities that stimulate, challenge, and increase blood flow to the brain. Cognitive abilities include:

■ Memory and communication skills.

■ Attention and concentration.

■ Perception—how the brain interprets information received from the senses.

■ Visuo-spatial awareness—how your brain interprets visual information and spatial relationships.

■ Executive functions, such as thinking, reasoning, decision-making, determining risk, and recognizing the impact that you have on others.

▲ Enjoying creative pursuits may boost your well-being and confidence. Some people feel it also improves their cognitive ability.

■ Gross-motor skills—controlling your body to make larger movements such as walking.

■ Fine-motor skills—controlling your body to make small movements such as manipulating a pen.

Mood and behavior

Your hobbies and interests help to shape you as a person and if you stop doing the things you enjoy, you may become depressed, stressed, or anxious. If you struggle to express those feelings, you might appear to be more quick-tempered to people around you. Meaningful activities will help you to feel more in control of yourself and your life.

Get the balance right

This book slots activities into three categories: self-care, productivity, and leisure. Some activities will fall under more than one category, depending on your likes and dislikes, but it is important that you get a balance of activities in your life in order to maintain your physical and mental health.

Finding balance

These categories are not rigid—for example, taking part in a yoga class could be leisure, but it is also a way of taking care of yourself. The important thing is to include activities that strike a balance between self-care, productivity, and leisure, so that you can find those that best suit your personal preferences.

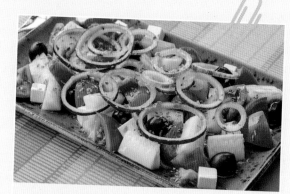

Productivity
Doing something useful may help you maintain your sense of self-worth. Productivity includes all activities where you produce something, such as making a meal, planting a container, or planning an outing.

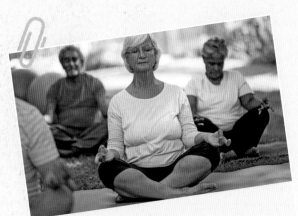

Self-care activities
These are the things we do each day to care for ourselves, such as eating, cleaning our home, and taking medication. Looking after yourself physically and mentally also falls under self-care.

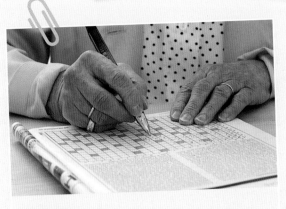

Leisure
Leisure activities are the things you do in your spare time, such as going on outings, engaging in hobbies, spending time with others, reading a book, or doing a crossword puzzle.

Which activity is right for me?

It is impossible to dictate which activities are going to be right for you, as people have different likes and interests. To stay motivated and get the most from activities, choose ones that you enjoy and that interest you. Keep doing the things you have always done, to the best of your ability. If things are becoming more difficult for you, you need to choose a level of activity that suits your current ability (a practice known as "grading").

Be prepared to share

You could seek support and assistance with the things you are struggling with. Sharing activities in this way can help you to continue doing the things that give you pleasure. You may also find that the people around you take over some of the everyday activities. However, if you are to maintain the skills you have, you need to practice them as much as you can.

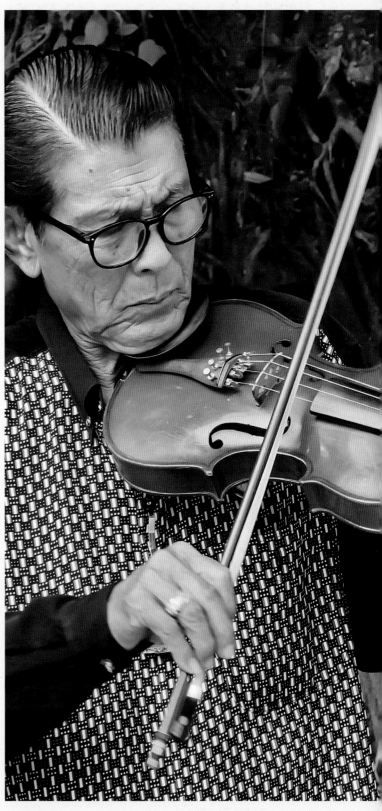

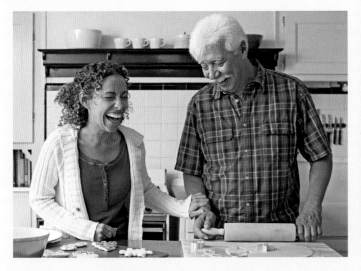

▲ Cooking and baking could be seen as a productive activity that also is part of self-care, but if it is your hobby, it also counts as leisure. It is also a good activity to share with someone else.

▲ Don't be discouraged when things become more difficult. Even an accomplished violinist couldn't play a demanding piece well without rehearsing it. We all need to practice skills to maintain them.

Make your life manageable

As your abilities change, you may have to adapt some of your activities, or break down activities into smaller tasks, so you can continue to take part. Match each activity to your current skills and abilities.

Adapting activities

If you're beginning to struggle with some meaningful activities, you may consider adapting them to meet your changing abilities. Choose a level of activity that suits you. The key to success is ensuring that you neither overestimate your ability and attempt activities that are too challenging, nor underestimate your ability and become frustrated.

Break it down

To adapt activities to ensure that they are just right for you, it is important that you have a true sense of the steps involved in completing them. It is easy to underestimate the complexity of some activities because you will be used to doing many of them each day without having to think about it. One way of understanding this is to think about a recipe, for example a recipe for making a sandwich. The recipe would tell you the equipment you would need, the ingredients required,

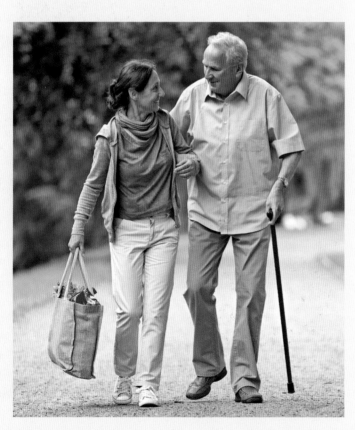

▲ If you can no longer walk without the use of a cane, consider taking someone with you when you go shopping to help carry your groceries.

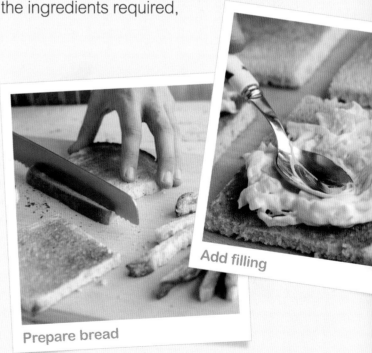

Add filling

Prepare bread

▲ Break down activities into manageable steps and then follow the sequence so that something seemingly complicated becomes easy.

TALK ABOUT...

Your favorite things to do outdoors

Do you enjoy making food or is it a chore?

How many steps are there to making a cup of coffee?

How does it work

If you are an avid baker, but are now unable to follow complex recipes, it does not mean you will never bake again. Simplify the recipe by breaking it down into easy steps. You may be able to share the activity with another person and do only the parts you feel

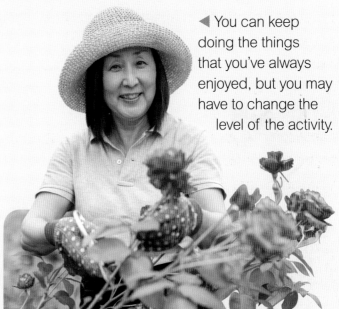

◀ You can keep doing the things that you've always enjoyed, but you may have to change the level of the activity.

and the step-by-step instructions of what you need to do. Most activities can be broken down into a recipe in the same way. Break down everyday activities—such as making a cup of coffee, brushing your teeth, mowing the lawn, or playing a card game—into smaller steps to find the recipe for each of them. This breakdown of steps provides you with all the information you require to successfully complete the activity.

comfortable doing. If you have always enjoyed gardening, you may not want to tidy hedges with an electric hedge trimmer, but may still enjoy pruning the roses, growing vegetables, or raking leaves. With this approach, you can continue to do the things you have always done and enjoyed, in a way that ensures success. Taking part in the activity is more important than the end result.

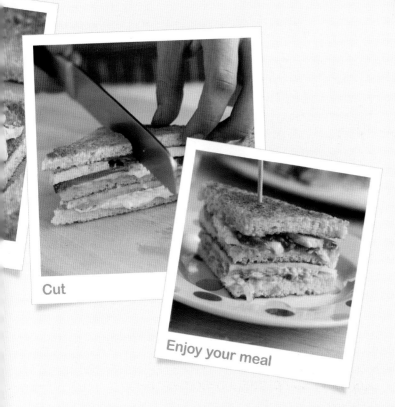

Cut

Enjoy your meal

How to use the activities in this book

There is growing evidence that being physically, mentally, and socially active may help maintain brain health. Using your existing skills and compensating for any difficulties you experience may help to slow the progression of dementia. In this book, there is a broad range of activities to help you sustain a healthy and balanced life.

Choosing activities

Each chapter includes the guidelines for different activities to meet a range of different abilities. Some activities may be too complex, while others may seem too easy. Try to find activities that match your current level of ability and skill and that appeal to you from each chapter. Activities need to be challenging enough that you get a sense of achievement from them, but not so difficult that you become frustrated by them, or give up.

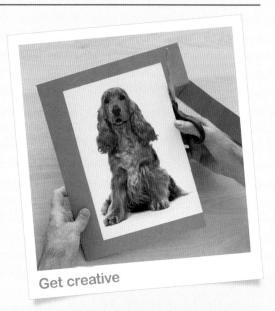

Get creative

Family and friends

A lot of the activities in this book can be enjoyed together with family or friends. Another person may do part of the activity, while you do another, or you may do it together. For example, if you enjoy baking or woodworking, but lack the confidence to use some of the appliances or tools, share the activity with someone else who can do the things you're less confident about. You don't have to rule out any activity altogether, and sharing activities also helps to keep you socially engaged and connected.

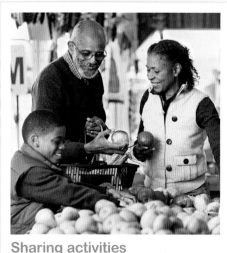

Sharing activities

Right thing, right time

Some people feel more alert and better able to concentrate in the morning; others prefer to be more active in the afternoon. Try to fit your activities around the times that suit you best. For example, if you are going swimming, it may be worth checking beforehand to find out when the pool is likely to be quiet. You may need to be flexible. If you planned an outdoor excursion for a particular day and wake up to pouring rain, or are not feeling at your best, it may be wise to postpone it for another time.

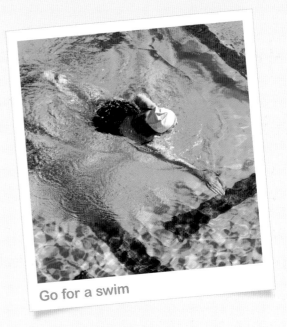
Go for a swim

Plan for the future

Some activities in this book may benefit you at a later stage in your dementia, such as making a sensory blanket, a fidget cuff, or memory cards and signs. You may not need the signs now, but they may help to alleviate disorientation later on. Establishing a household routine now may help you handle doing an activity longer. Get into the habit of using a calendar or always putting any appointment reminders on a bulletin board.

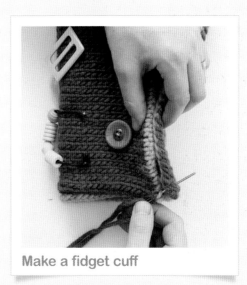
Make a fidget cuff

Activity pages

This book is filled with stimulating activities to keep you busy. For each activity, you are told how difficult it is, the time it takes to complete it, the category it falls in (self-care, productivity, or leisure), and the reasons that activity may be good for you. Potential safety issues have also been identified. Use these guidelines to choose activities that suit you best. There are talking points on many pages, posing questions or helping you to think more widely about the topic.

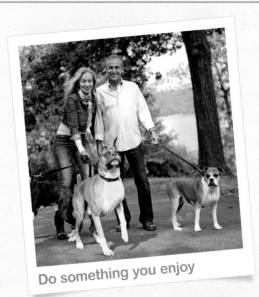
Do something you enjoy

OUT
AND
ABOUT

It is important for your physical and mental health to keep active and involved with the world outside your home. Physical activity of any kind—from doing sports or gardening, to taking a walk in the park or shopping—may help keep you strong, supple, and more alert. It can also improve your memory, appetite, and quality of sleep. Simply being outdoors can lift your spirits and make you feel good about yourself. Sharing activities with family and friends is best of all to keep you connected and avoid isolation.

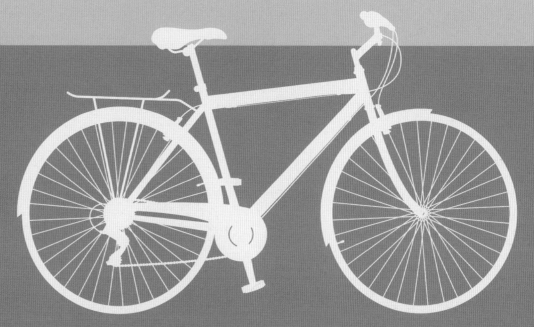

Aerobic exercise

Any exercise that increases heart and breathing rates, and oxygen circulation in your blood, is aerobic. It benefits the mind, body, and soul.

How to do it

There are many aerobic activities, such as swimming, riding a bike, or engaging in team sports. Choose one that you enjoy.

■ Take regular rest breaks and drink plenty of fluids to stay hydrated. Refuel with healthy snacks.

■ Build aerobic exercise into everyday activities such as walking the dog and doing household chores.

■ Don't overdo it: you should be able to talk while exercising.

■ Even going up and down the stairs frequently helps physical fitness, mobility, and balance.

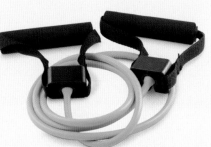

▲ Combine aerobic exercise with resistance training, using weights, exercise bands, or even gravity.

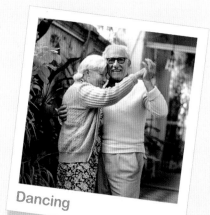

Dancing

What have you always done to keep fit?
•
Have you ever used a celebrity's exercise video to make exercising more interesting?
•
Which do you like best—watching sports or taking part?

TALK ABOUT...

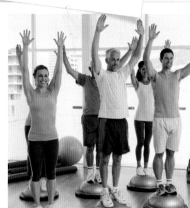

Group classes

AT A GLANCE

✓ Active to gentle activity

✓ 1 or more people

✓ Self-care/leisure

✓ Variable timeframe

✓ Variable difficulty

! Talk to your doctor before beginning any exercise program

HOW IT HELPS

People over age 50 who do 45–60 minutes of moderate aerobic exercise on most days show improved cognition.

• Brain function may improve, which may slow down memory loss and enhance mental flexibility, working memory, and self-control.

• Aerobic exercise helps heart health, bone strength, mobility, flexibilty, and overall fitness.

• Quality of sleep may improve.

• Aerobic exercise releases endorphins (feel-good hormones) that can improve your mood.

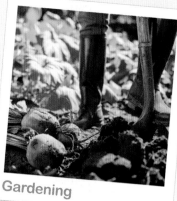

Gardening

◀ There are many forms of aerobic exercise; join a group or gym or practice on your own.

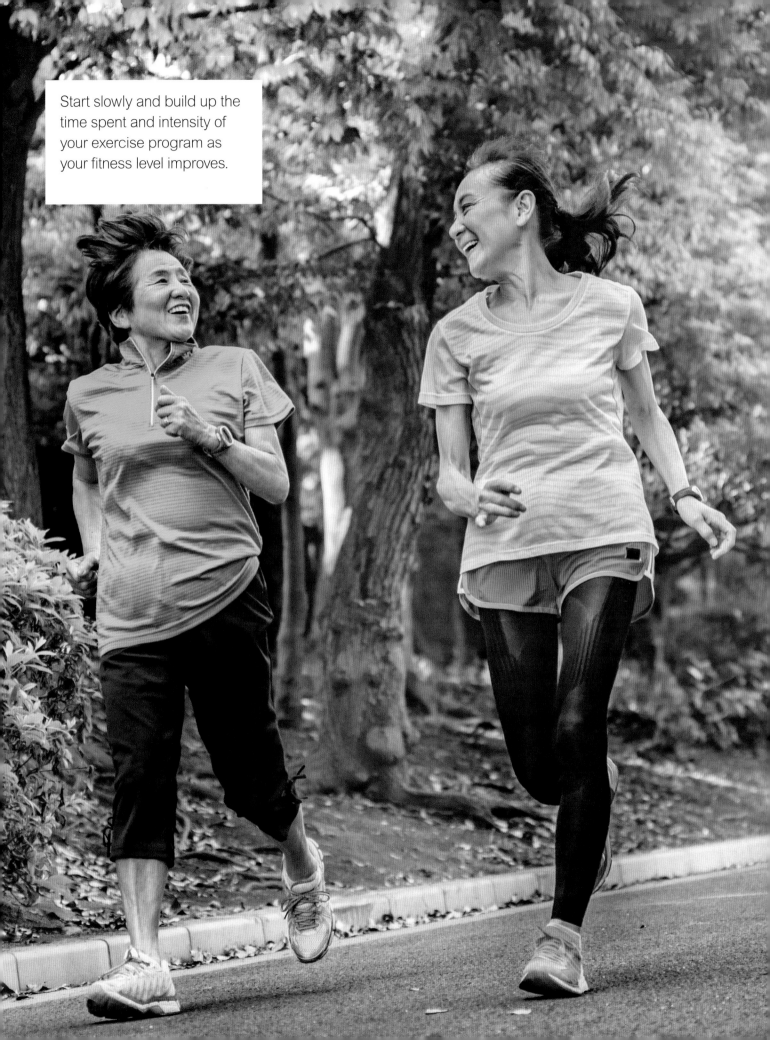

Start slowly and build up the time spent and intensity of your exercise program as your fitness level improves.

Ride a bike

If you have a passion for biking and want to continue enjoying it, there are some simple ways of adapting this activity to your ability.

How to do it

Plan your bike ride carefully and, if you're biking on roads, be aware of road safety.

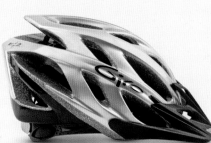

▲ Wear a helmet, reflective clothing, and suitable footwear.

■ Make sure you know your route and take a map; a GPS app on your cell phone can help with navigational difficulties and track your route.

■ Try joining a local bicycle club that has instructors on hand to guide and assist you.

■ Build in rest breaks; take plenty of water to keep you hydrated and some snacks for energy.

AT A GLANCE

✓ Active

✓ 1 or more people

✓ Leisure

✓ Variable timeframe

✓ Variable difficulty

! Be aware of road safety

! Talk to your doctor before beginning any exercise program

HOW IT HELPS

Biking combines the benefits of doing aerobics and being outdoors, so it is a good way to maintain physical fitness.

• If you have ridden a bike in the past, you should have a procedural memory of this skill.

• Biking maintains gross motor skills—mobility, flexibility, strength, and balance.

• Traveling by bike strengthens and uses many cognitive skills, including concentration and decision making.

• Biking releases endorphins (feel-good hormones that boost mental health and well-being).

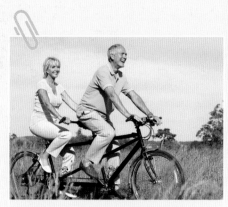

Different bicycles
If you are struggling on two wheels, try a tandem with someone or an adult tricycle.

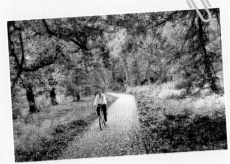

Choose a safe route
Wherever possible, use a flat, quiet path or back street rather than riding on a busy road.

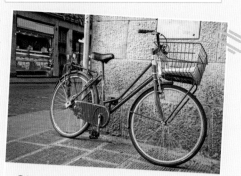

Short, local trips
Use local outings, like going to the store, as a chance to bike along a familiar route.

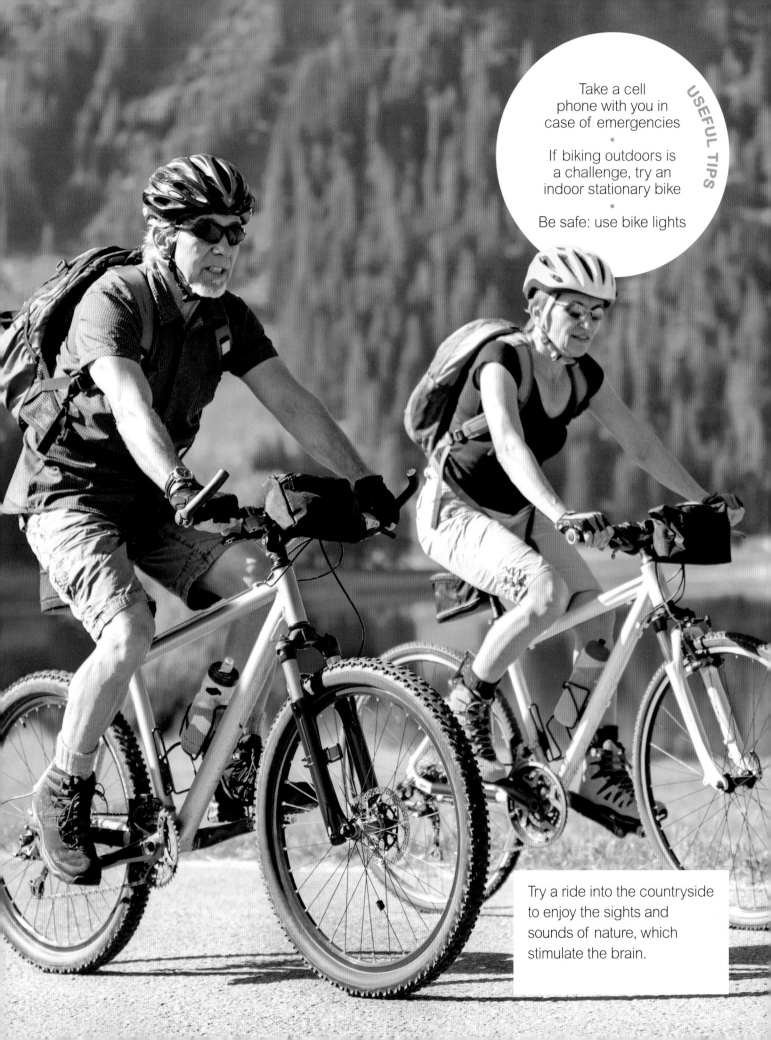

USEFUL TIPS

Take a cell phone with you in case of emergencies

•

If biking outdoors is a challenge, try an indoor stationary bike

•

Be safe: use bike lights

Try a ride into the countryside to enjoy the sights and sounds of nature, which stimulate the brain.

Go swimming

Swimming is a low-impact form of aerobic exercise and an ideal way of helping to maintain overall physical fitness and mental health.

How to do it

You might feel more confident taking someone with you to help navigate the changing rooms and to find out where everything is, especially if it is your first time.

■ Avoid busy times, such as mother and toddler sessions.

■ Make sure the pool is easily accessible, with ramps, wide steps, and ladders. Clear signage; softer, less reflective lighting; and easily accessible toilets also help.

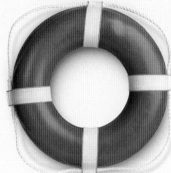

▲ If you have limitations, let the lifeguard know so they can keep an eye on you.

AT A GLANCE

✓ Active—low impact

✓ 1 or more people

✓ Self-care/leisure

✓ Variable timeframe

✓ Variable difficulty

! Be aware of water safety

! Talk to your doctor before beginning any exercise program

HOW IT HELPS

The buoyancy of water reduces any impact on bones and joints— which is especially good if you have conditions such as arthritis or any balance problems.

• The increased blood flow helps to promote heart health and may help brain function.

• This activity can decrease your risk of falling by strengthening the muscles needed for balance.

• Swimming helps relax the body and mind, reducing stress and anxiety and improving cognition.

• Swimming can boost your mood, positivity, and well-being, and promote deeper sleep.

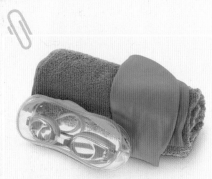

The correct equipment
Pack a bag with a swimsuit, towel, water shoes, goggles, and any other clothes, toiletries, and equipment you will need.

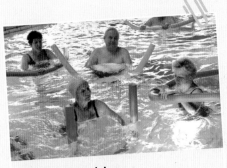

Water aerobics
Try water aerobics: water provides resistance to movement, making any exercise more effective.

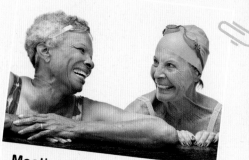

Meeting friends
The pool can be a place to relax, exercise, and meet new friends.

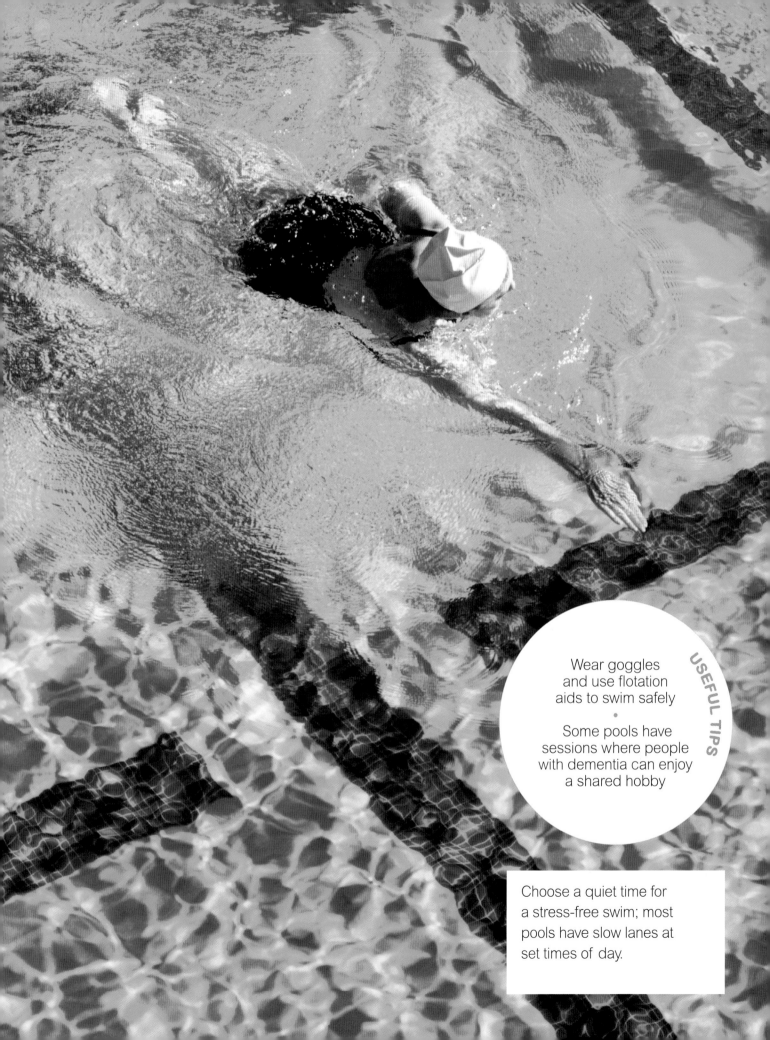

USEFUL TIPS

Wear goggles
and use flotation
aids to swim safely

Some pools have
sessions where people
with dementia can enjoy
a shared hobby

Choose a quiet time for
a stress-free swim; most
pools have slow lanes at
set times of day.

Sports heroes

Sports give people the opportunity to test their strength and skill against other athletes. With improved technology, records are constantly being broken, but true sports heroes are bound to be remembered.

Are you a fan or have you played a sport yourself?

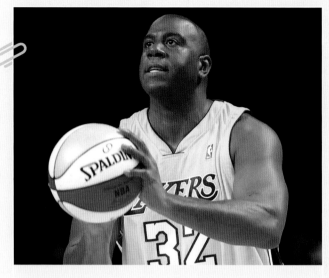

Basketball
Earvin "Magic" Johnson is a legendary basketball star who played for the Los Angeles Lakers and won a gold medal at the 1992 Olympic Games.

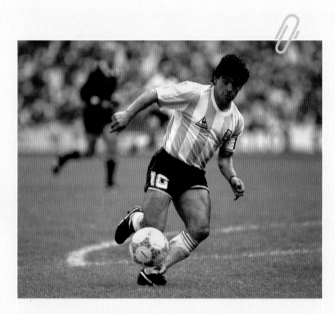

Soccer
Diego Maradona led the Argentinian team to win the 1986 World Cup and was voted joint FIFA Player of the 20th Century with the Brazilian Pelé.

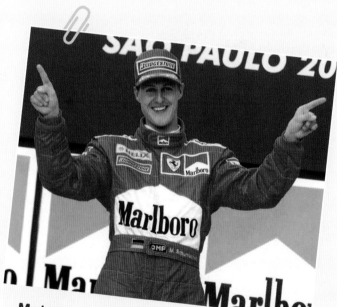

Motorsport
German race car driver Michael Schumacher is one of the most successful competitors in Formula One history. He won the Formula One World Drivers' Championship seven times.

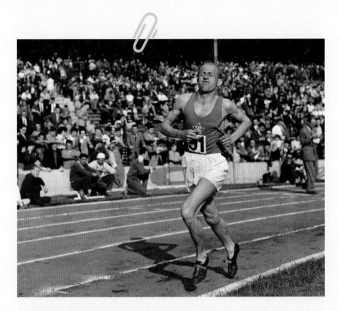

Track and Field
Czechoslovak Emil Zátopek (1922–2000) won three gold medals, for the 5,000 m, 10,000 m, and men's marathon in the 1952 Olympic Games.

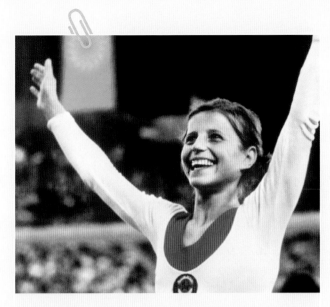

Gymnastics
At the age of 17, Olga Korbut won three gold medals and one silver medal as part of the Russian team in the 1972 Olympic Games in Munich.

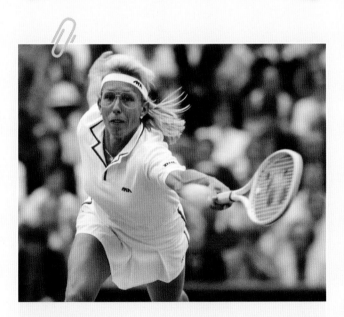

Tennis
Former world No. 1 singles and doubles player, Martina Navratilova won 59 Grand Slam titles: 18 singles, 31 doubles, and 10 mixed doubles.

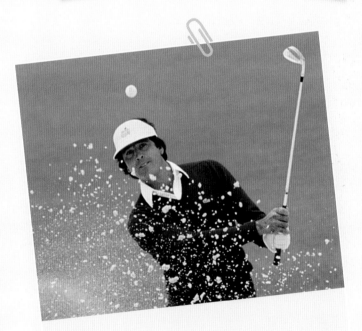

Golf
The Spanish golfer Severiano "Seve" Ballesteros (1957–2011) was one of the greats of the game, winning 5 majors and over 90 international tournaments.

Play a team sport

If you play a team sport, you can continue to enjoy the camaraderie and shared experience of your sport with some simple adaptations.

How to do it

If you have been a member of a team, but can no longer play, think of ways to continue to join in, rather than of reasons not to. The postgame talk will be the same.

■ Adapt the way you take part in the sport to suit you. For example, if you play golf, play nine holes rather than 18 and use a golf cart instead of walking the course.

■ Try a less active sport, such as horseshoes or bowling. Challenge family or friends to a game.

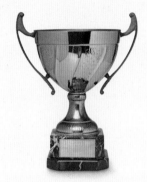

▲ If you have trophies from your sport, take them out and talk about them to friends and family.

HOW IT HELPS

Team sports, like all activities that combine physical, mental and social engagement, are most likely to slow cognitive decline in those living with dementia.

• Keeping physically fit and active may benefit brain function.

• Maintaining sports contacts and friendships may help to alleviate isolation and loneliness.

• Participation in a team sport can alleviate stress and depression, both of which exacerbate memory problems.

• Sharing a passion for sports provides opportunities for conversation and reminiscence.

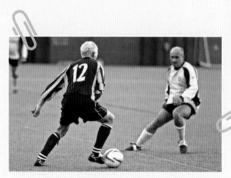

Veteran teams
Join a veteran team where the pace is slower, for example, walking soccer.

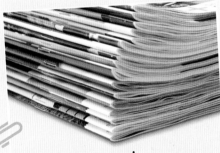

Follow your sport
Watch live events or classic recordings on TV or online, or look at books and magazines.

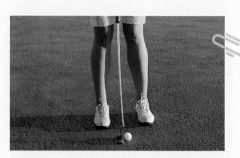

Find ways to keep playing
Instead of a full golf round, practice on a putting green or driving range.

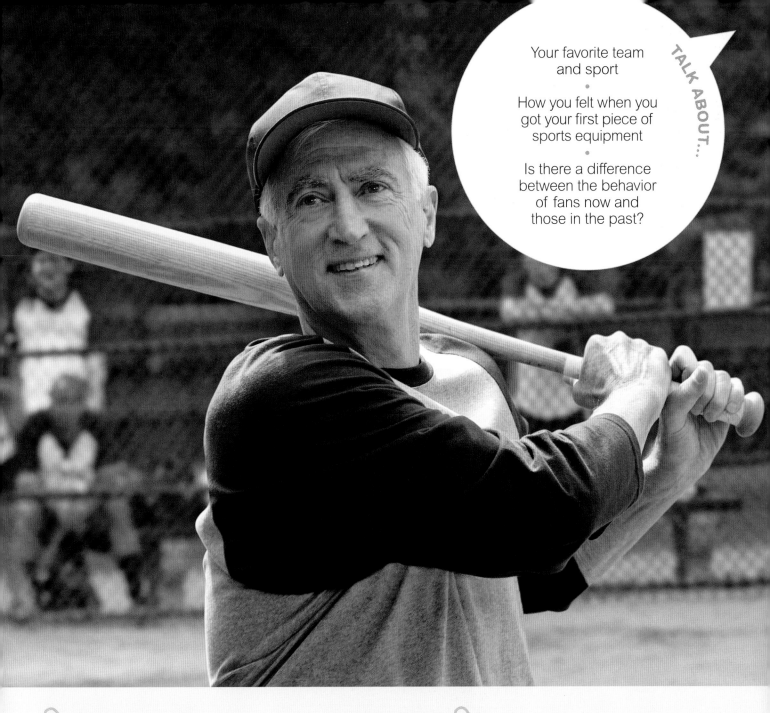

TALK ABOUT...

Your favorite team and sport

·

How you felt when you got your first piece of sports equipment

·

Is there a difference between the behavior of fans now and those in the past?

▲ Keep playing for as long as you can. Try to find a local team that plays at a level that is challenging, but not so challenging that you don't enjoy it.

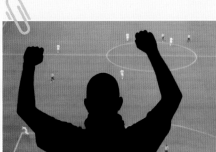

Be a supporter
Be an active supporter, by watching games and joining a fan club.

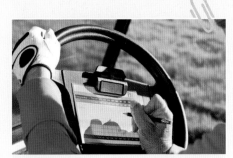

Get a teammate to help
Get help from a teammate with the challenging parts of your sport, like keeping score.

Keep strong and supple

Many gentler forms of exercise, from a walk to low-impact sports or fitness classes, help you to stay strong and supple.

How to do it

Consider exercising with a family member or friend, or as part of group. Often this can be more fun and helps to motivate you to keep going.

■ Local fitness centers often run classes to help mature adults to improve strength and balance. Instructors are trained to adapt activities and modify exercises to accommodate any issues you may have.

■ Wear comfortable clothing and suitable footwear.

■ Take a drink and a snack with you.

TALK ABOUT...
Pros and cons of martial arts

•

Other things that keep you fit, such as walking the dog, doing housework, and going up stairs

•

Your favorite kung fu artist

AT A GLANCE

✓ Active

✓ 1 or more people

✓ Self-care/leisure

✓ Variable timeframe

✓ Moderate difficulty

! Talk to your doctor before beginning any exercise program

HOW IT HELPS

Even gentle exercise releases endorphins into the bloodstream, improving mood and confidence.

• Exercises that improve balance, coordination, flexibility, and strength also ease pain and stiffness and reduce falling risks.

• Some exercises involve deep breathing, which has a calming effect, reducing stress and anxiety.

• Following an exercise class demands cognitive skills such as remembering sequences and understanding instructions.

• Exercising in a group encourages social interaction and communication skills.

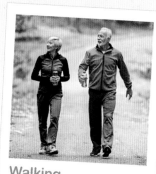
Walking

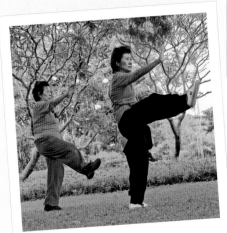
Tai chi

▲ Try different activities to find one that suits you best. Many classes allow you to attend a trial session.

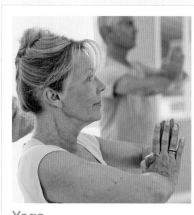
Yoga

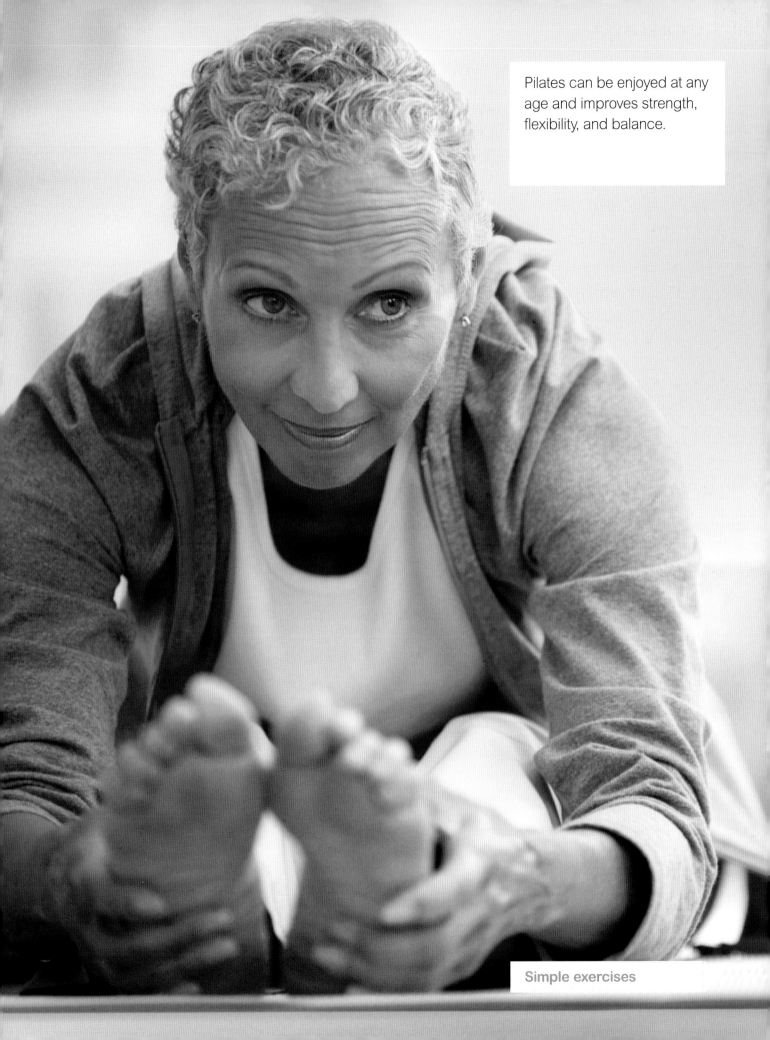

Pilates can be enjoyed at any age and improves strength, flexibility, and balance.

Simple exercises

Simple exercises

If you find it difficult to get up and move around, here are some simple exercises you can do at home.

■ Wear comfortable clothes and, if needed, appropriate footwear.

■ Warm up gently and work at your own pace. You should be able to talk while exercising and not struggle for breath. If you feel pain or discomfort, stop.

■ Try a range of different exercises.

■ Be sure to cool down after exercising.

AT A GLANCE

✓ Active

✓ 1 or more people

✓ Self-care

✓ Little and often

✓ Easy

! Talk to your doctor before beginning any exercise program

◄ Bottled water, small beanbags, canned food, or a lightweight ball make good homemade weights.

Building strength

Even small movements will build muscle strength. Try pushing against a wall, as in the example shown below.

WALL PRESS

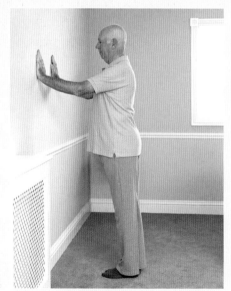 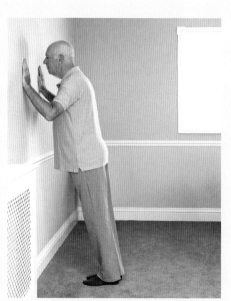 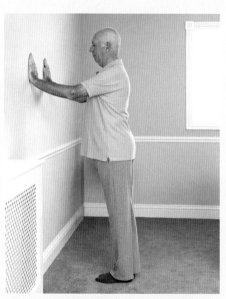

1 Place your palms at chest height against the wall, fingers pointing up, with hands just over shoulder-width apart and arms slightly bent.

2 Keeping your back straight, bend your elbows and slowly lean forward until your head is close to the wall. Your feet should not move.

3 Push against the wall and slowly return to the starting position, with your body upright. Repeat the push-up about 10 times if possible.

Armchair exercises

Try these exercises on your own or as part of a group. Choose a chair that is solid and stable. You should be able to sit upright with your knees at right angles and feet flat.

TALK ABOUT...

What are you: a couch potato or gym bunny?

Good music to exercise to

Describe your usual fitness routine

SQUATS

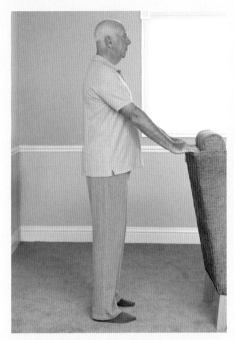 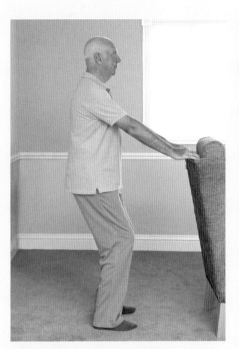 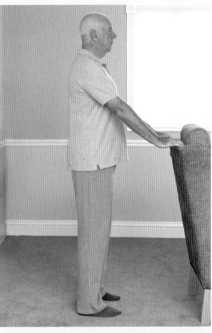

1 Hold on to the back of a stable chair for support, if you feel the need to. Stand straight with your feet about hip-width apart.

2 Keeping your back straight, gently bend your knees. Keep looking forward. Lower your body only as far as is comfortable.

3 Return to a standing position and repeat the squat 5 times if possible. Do an extra squat each time you do the exercise until you can do 10.

FOOT WALK

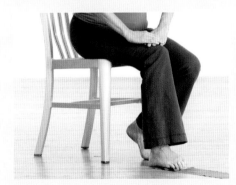 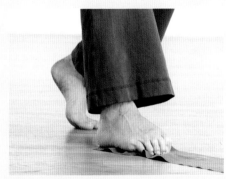 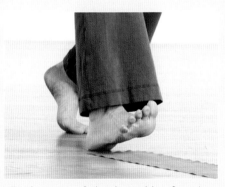

1 Use a chair that allows you to sit with your feet flat on the floor. Spread an exercise band or dish towel on the floor with one end under your foot.

2 Pull the band toward your heel by gripping it with your toes, and then curling the arch of your foot to gather up a small amount of the band.

3 Let go of the band by fanning out your toes. Repeat until you reach the end of the band. Spread it out under the other foot and repeat the exercise.

Simple relaxation routines

Making relaxation a part of your daily routine allows you to have a break from the stresses of everyday life, which may help brain health.

How to do it

There are many different types of relaxation exercises, including visualization, mindfulness, and simple muscle relaxation. Choose a relaxation method that works for you and try to make time for it every day.

■ Visualization is a process where you close your eyes and imagine yourself in a special place—such as on a mountain, by a stream, on a beach, or in a garden. Concentrate on what you can "see" in that place, and how that makes you feel.

■ Mindfulness is about being in the moment: concentrate on yourself, your breathing and senses, and reconnect with your surroundings.

■ Simple muscle relaxation involves contracting and then relaxing different muscle groups.

AT A GLANCE

✓ Sedentary

✓ 1 person

✓ 1–30 minutes

✓ Moderate difficulty

✓ Self-care

HOW IT HELPS

Relaxation is not the same as just resting. Having the opportunity to relax each day allows you to quiet your thoughts, reducing stress, and improving your overall sense of well-being.

● Physically relaxing the muscles and breathing more deeply and slowly increases blood flow to the brain, making you more alert.

● Relaxing can help you feel more motivated and productive.

● It has been found to benefit people who experience agitation as a symptom of a dementia by reducing anxiety.

● Relaxation can also reduce physical aches and relieve pain.

● It improves sleep, but relaxation is not about sleeping.

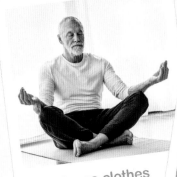

Wear loose clothes

Put your feet up

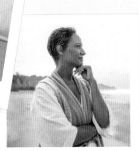

Find a quiet place

TALK ABOUT…

Where do you feel most relaxed?

Have you used any particular relaxation methods before?

▲ Choose a time and place where you won't be disturbed, and get comfortable.

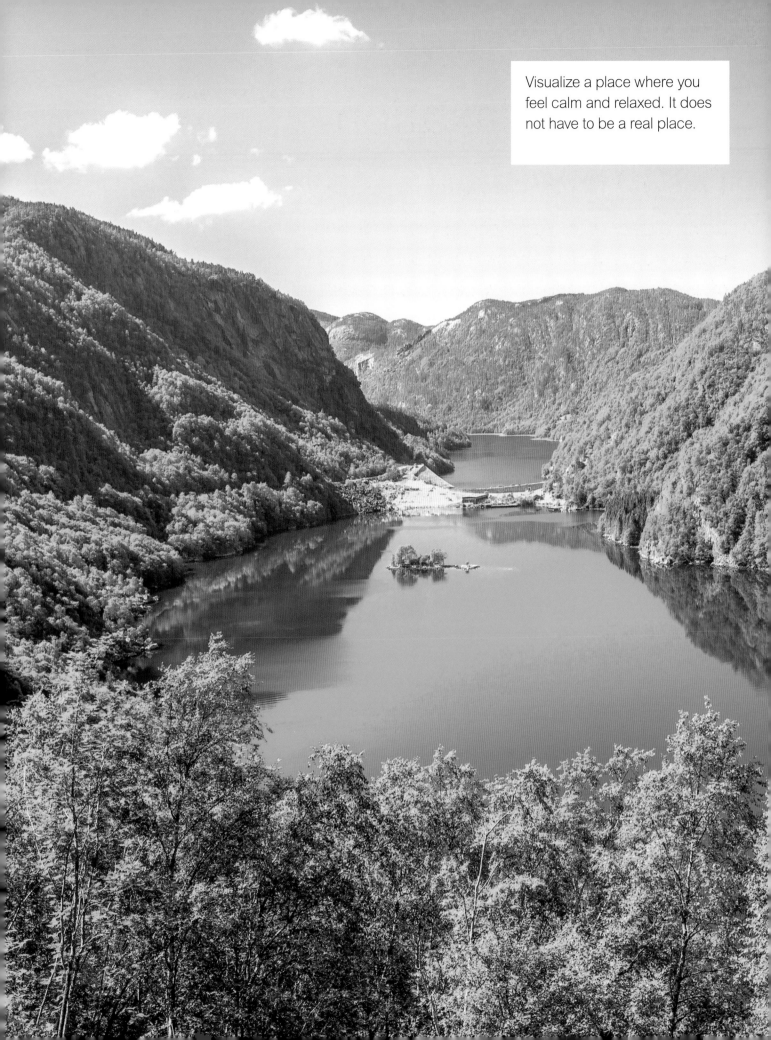

Visualize a place where you feel calm and relaxed. It does not have to be a real place.

Go on a nature walk

Being outdoors and connecting with nature is known as "green exercise." It is a chance to revisit favorite places or explore new ones either on your own, with friends, or in a group.

How to do it

Walking with others can be fun and may make you feel safer; perhaps you could join a walking group.

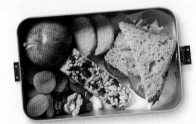

▲ Include rest breaks—stop at a coffee shop on the way, or pack a picnic.

■ Start slowly and increase the difficulty as your fitness and mobility improves. A walk in the local park may suit you better than a mountain hike!

■ If going alone, tell someone where you are going and what time you plan to be back and take a cell phone; some phones have apps that can track your route.

■ Plan your route well and check the weather forecast. Put on your walking shoes, and go!

AT A GLANCE

✓ Active

✓ 1 or more people

✓ Leisure

✓ Variable timeframe

✓ Choose a route to match your fitness level

! Take a drink and a snack. If going alone, think about personal safety

HOW IT HELPS

Green exercise has extra value for those living with dementia, as well as raising vitamin D levels (good for bone health and mood).

• Walking helps you to sleep better and improves appetite.

• Green exercise may make it easier for you to express yourself verbally.

• A walk in nature provides sensory stimulation from all the things you see and do, and an opportunity for reminiscing.

• Some people find that being in nature makes their dementia symptoms less obvious, because there is less focus on them.

TALK ABOUT...

Do you prefer a mountain hike or countryside stroll?

•

What is your favorite season?

•

Do you like a warm day or cold, blustery day?

•

Who is your favorite adventurer?

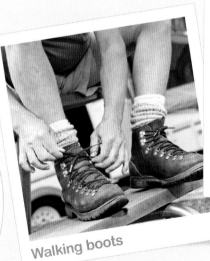

Walking boots

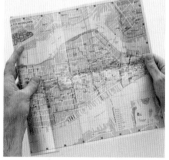

Take a map

▲ Think about taking a map and compass, and wear suitable clothing.

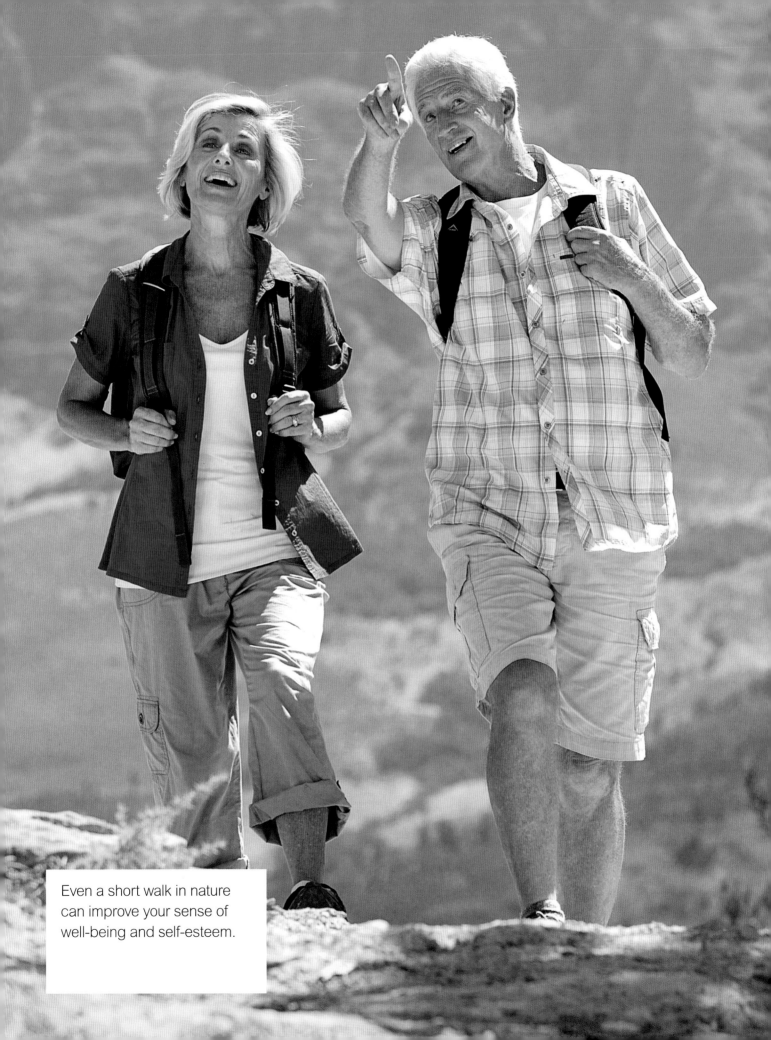

Even a short walk in nature can improve your sense of well-being and self-esteem.

Keep a nature diary

Whether you go on a nature walk, sit in your garden, or simply look out of the window, keeping a nature diary helps you to appreciate the natural environment.

How to do it

Decide what to include in the diary. Do you want to record each nature walk or focus on a theme, such as trees or wildlife?

■ You could compare the seasons by visiting the same locations at different times of year.

■ Record your thoughts, feelings, and observations at the time. Be as descriptive as possible and include any questions to explore later.

■ You could record your observations in a notebook or as a voice memo on your cell phone, and take photos or make sketches.

▶ Collect interesting or beautiful items that you spot along the way. They need to be fairly flat and small to fit in a diary.

AT A GLANCE

✓ Active/sedentary

✓ 1 or more people

✓ Productivity

✓ No time limit

✓ Easy

HOW IT HELPS

This project focuses your concentration and encourages you to be more active.

• Looking for material to include in a nature diary exercises observational skills.

• You can use all of your senses to appreciate the natural world around you.

• Smell is the most powerful trigger of emotional memory, because that sense is strongly connected to the memory and emotion centers of the brain.

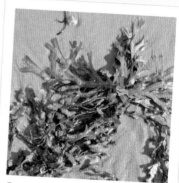

Seaweed

Leaves

TALK ABOUT...

What are your favorite childhood memories of being in nature?

•

Are insects valuable?

•

Where do you feel most at home in nature?

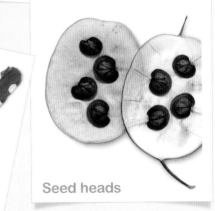

Feathers

Seed heads

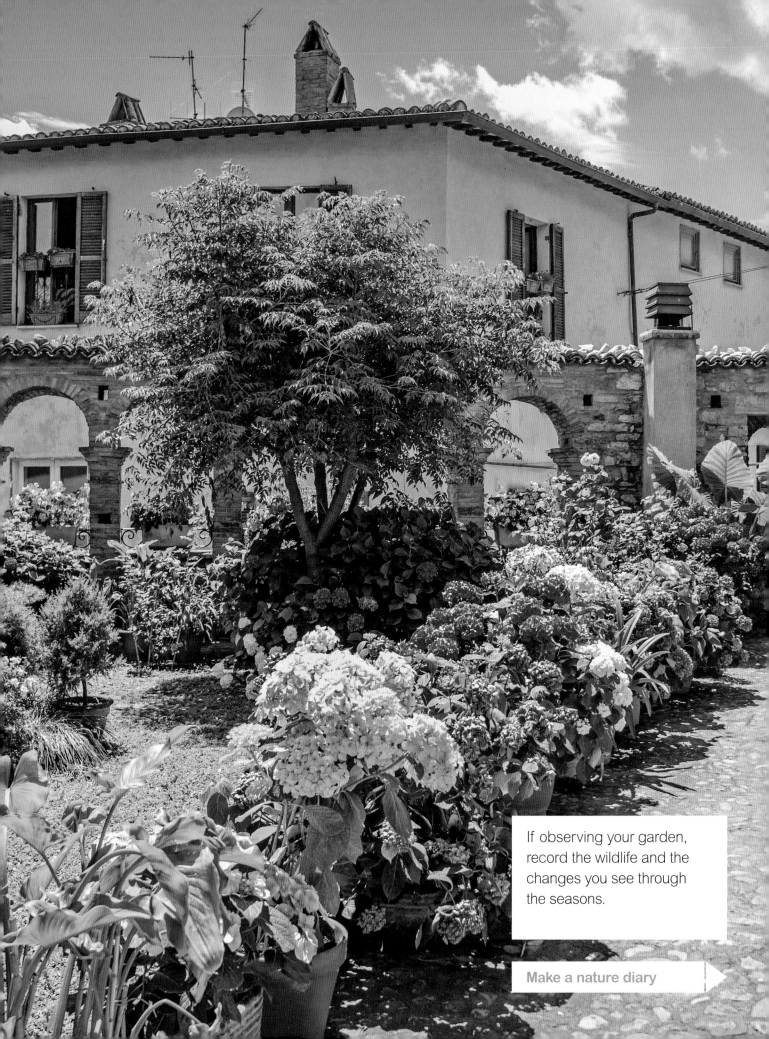

If observing your garden, record the wildlife and the changes you see through the seasons.

Make a nature diary ▷

Make a nature diary

This project will grow over time into your personal record of nature around you. It can be as simple or as detailed as you wish.

How to do it

Start by choosing a book, such as a scrapbook or large notebook, for your nature diary and think how you will capture the information.

■ Organize your workspace so that everything you need is handy, where you can see it. A contrasting cloth, especially red, underneath the materials helps with visual perception.

■ Before putting items in your diary, arrange them on the page first. This way you can be sure there is plenty of space for everything and that you have left enough room to make notes.

USEFUL TIPS

Research, in books or online, the names of plants and animals you've seen

•

Complete your diary pages regularly to avoid difficulty in identifying and collating items

AT A GLANCE

✓ Gentle activity/sedentary

✓ 1 or more people

✓ Productivity

✓ No time limit

✓ Easy

HOW IT HELPS

The diary will provide a record to aid your memory recall when sharing your findings with others.

• Planning and organizing your diary involves the front part of the brain—the executive management center.

• You will use visuo-spatial skills and hand-eye coordination to lay out the pages.

• Being creative can help with making decisions and positively influences well-being.

▲ Don't pick wildflowers or their seed heads, photograph or draw them instead.

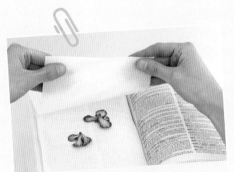

Press plant material
Press flowers or leaves between paper towels inside a book for about four weeks.

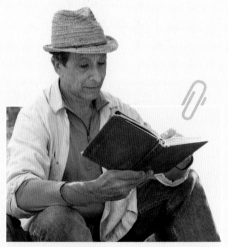

Draw or paint
If you like drawing or painting, record views or details of animals or plants.

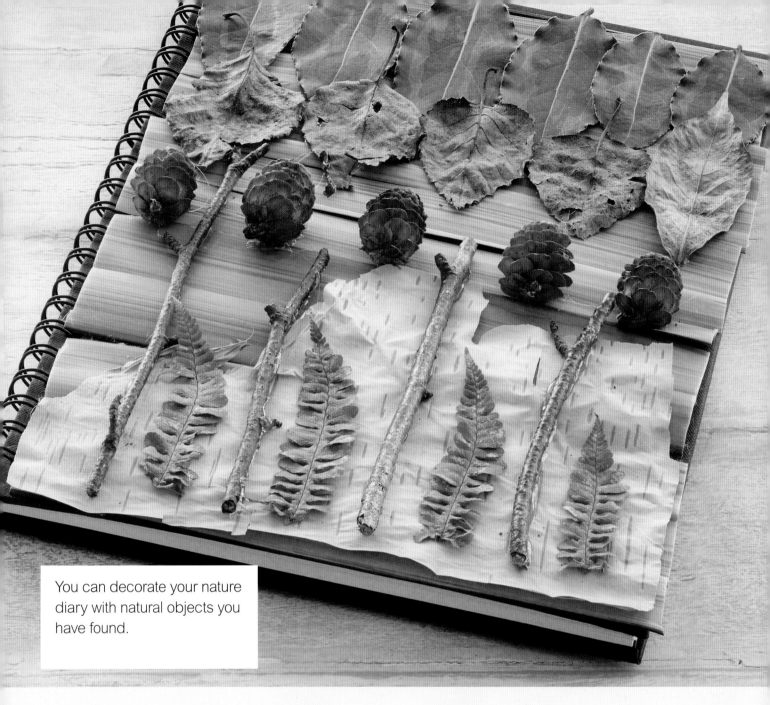

You can decorate your nature diary with natural objects you have found.

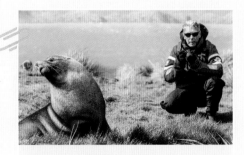

Take a photograph
Photograph what you see: scenery, wildlife, or details such as bird tracks or wildflowers.

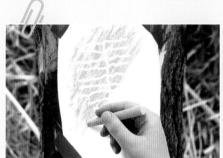

Take a bark rubbing
Tape paper to a tree trunk and use a soft crayon to capture an interesting bark pattern.

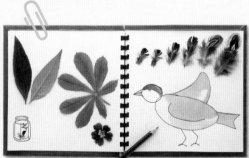

Compile your diary
Paste or tape each memento in the diary with a note of the place, date, time, and weather.

Walk the dog

For many people, walking the dog is one of the great pleasures of life. It gets you out and about in all weather and gives you a chance to be sociable.

How to do it

Plan your route carefully, taking into account your general fitness, weather conditions, and time of day.

▲ Pack everything you need (cell phone, money, keys, a drink, a leash, dog treats, and poop bags).

■ It is generally best to stick to familiar routes.

■ If you don't own a dog, borrow one or go with a friend who has one.

■ If going alone, consider your safety. Having a GPS app on your cell phone is useful.

HOW IT HELPS

Walking the dog improves your overall fitness, heart health, muscle strength, and bone density. It may also improve brain function, slowing down the effects of memory impairment.

• This activity can help you feel oriented and maintain cognitive skills such as planning, organizing, as well as initiating and completing tasks.

• Petting your dog lowers the stress hormone, cortisol. Lifelike model dogs can have the same effect.

• Dogs spark conversation with passersby, bringing a social element to the activity and helping to reduce the risk of loneliness.

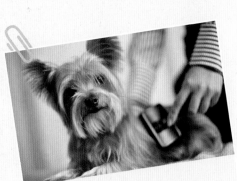

Groom your dog
Brushing your dog after a walk is good for it and for you; it reduces stress and improves your mood.

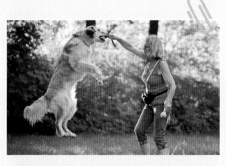

Play with your dog
If you can walk only a short distance, exercise the dog—and your coordination—by throwing toys for it to fetch.

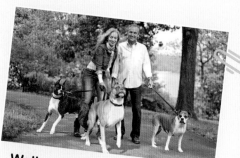

Walk with friends
Join a dog-walking group to share experiences and to reduce the risk of losing your way.

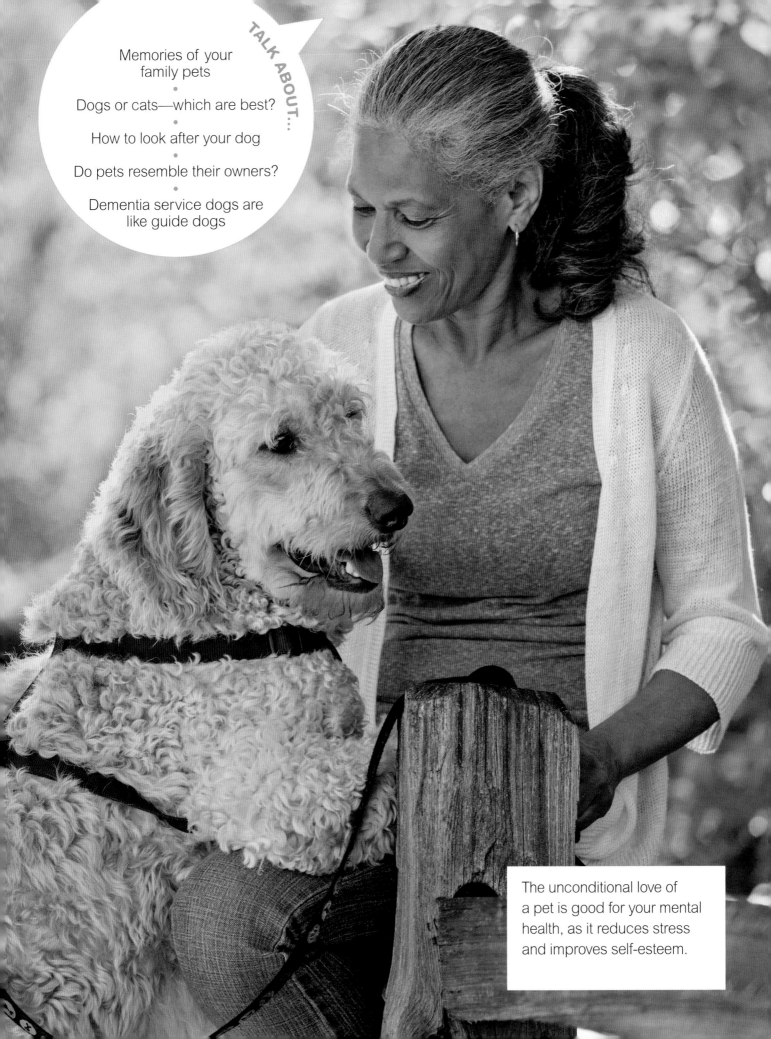

TALK ABOUT...

Memories of your
family pets

•

Dogs or cats—which are best?

•

How to look after your dog

•

Do pets resemble their owners?

•

Dementia service dogs are
like guide dogs

The unconditional love of
a pet is good for your mental
health, as it reduces stress
and improves self-esteem.

Go shopping

Many people with dementia say shopping is their favorite activity. It can help keep you mentally and physically active and engaged with your local community.

How to do it

Loneliness has a negative impact on communication skills and mood. Going to the store each day, even to buy one item, could help you to feel less isolated.

■ Take time to check your cupboards to see what you need, then write a shopping list before you head out.

■ Be organized. Planning your trip carefully makes the shopping experience less stressful and more enjoyable.

■ Avoid busy times of the day, and look for larger stores with trained staff who can help you.

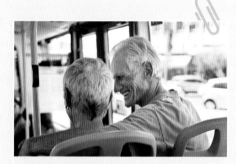

Transportation
It might be less tiring to choose stores that are a little farther away but nearer to the bus stop or parking lot.

AT A GLANCE

✓ Active

✓ 1 or more people

✓ Self-care

✓ Variable timeframe

✓ Variable difficulty

! Requires road-safety and money skills

HOW IT HELPS

Going to the store keeps you familiar with your local area and provides an opportunity to reminisce about how things have changed.

• Planning your route and your trip uses a range of cognitive skills.

• You use decision-making skills in choosing what to buy and where to find it.

• Managing money is often hard for people with dementia, even in the early days. Paying makes you use your working memory to do the math and handle bills and coins, so your confidence increases.

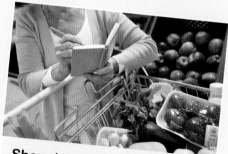

Shopping list
Taking a list of what you need can reduce the pressure to remember while you are at the store.

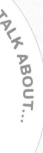

TALK ABOUT...

How has your main street changed?

•

Do you prefer local stores or large malls?

•

Have you tried online shopping?

•

What is your favorite type of store?

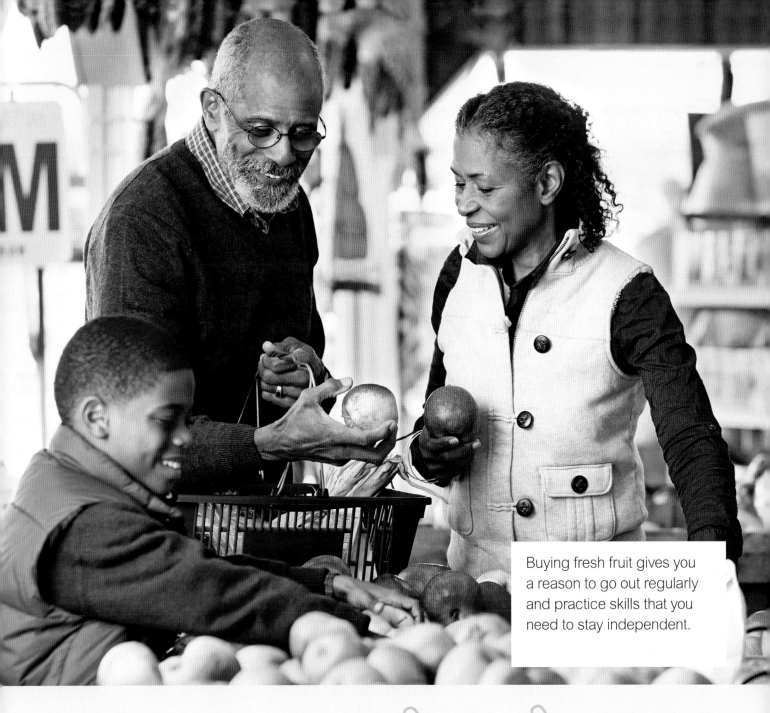

Buying fresh fruit gives you a reason to go out regularly and practice skills that you need to stay independent.

Shopping bags
If you need more items than you can easily carry, or need to use a cane, take someone with you to help out.

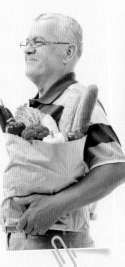

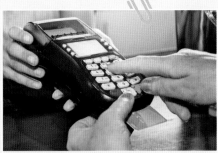

Paying
If dealing with cash is putting you off going shopping, use a credit or debit card instead.

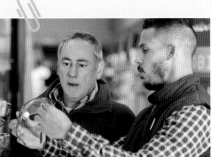

Asking for help
Asking a store clerk for help uses your social and decision-making skills.

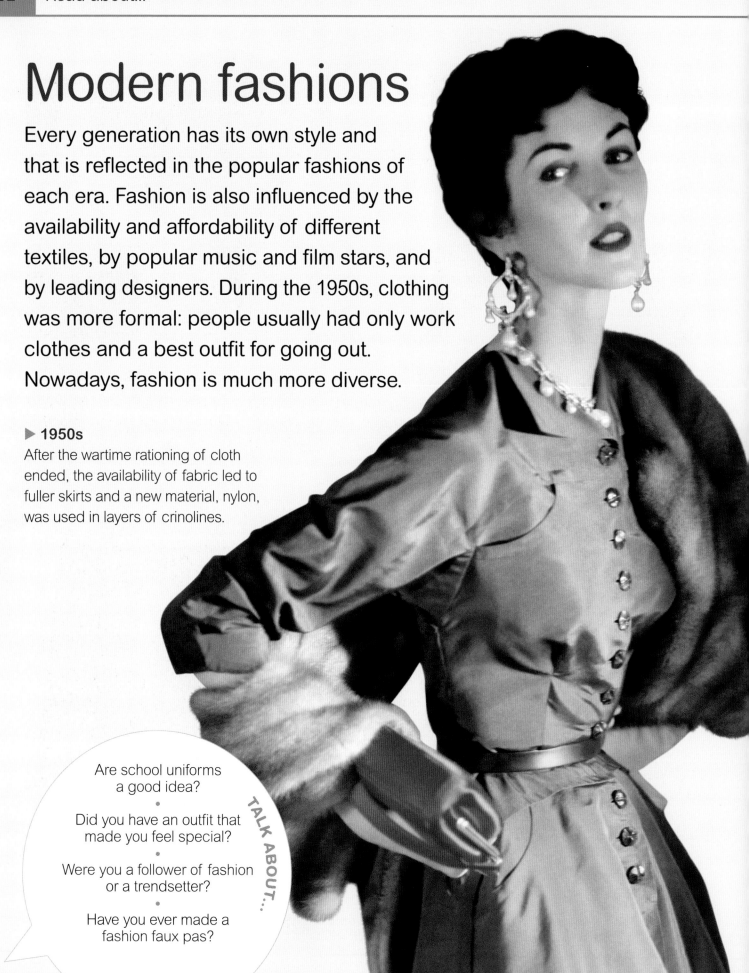

Modern fashions

Every generation has its own style and that is reflected in the popular fashions of each era. Fashion is also influenced by the availability and affordability of different textiles, by popular music and film stars, and by leading designers. During the 1950s, clothing was more formal: people usually had only work clothes and a best outfit for going out. Nowadays, fashion is much more diverse.

▶ **1950s**
After the wartime rationing of cloth ended, the availability of fabric led to fuller skirts and a new material, nylon, was used in layers of crinolines.

TALK ABOUT...

Are school uniforms
a good idea?
•
Did you have an outfit that
made you feel special?
•
Were you a follower of fashion
or a trendsetter?
•
Have you ever made a
fashion faux pas?

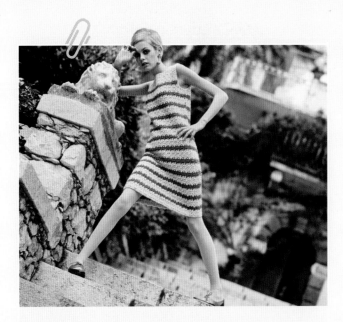

1960s

The early 1960s is synonymous with the miniskirt and minidress, as modeled by supermodel Twiggy. Dresses were form-fitting and often had geometric patterns.

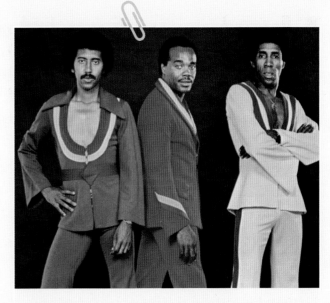

1970s

This decade saw the use of new synthetic materials in bright colors. The '70s look was defined by tight-fitting pants, tank tops, and platform shoes.

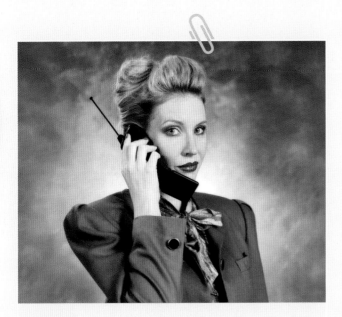

1980s

In this decade, "power dressing" became fashionable, when men and women wore tailored suits with big shoulder pads to show how successful they were.

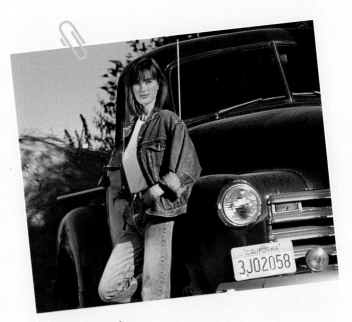

Modern day

Over the decades, denim jeans, T-shirts, and sneakers have evolved to become the accepted casual outfit for all generations across the world.

Go on an outing

An outing, whether to shop or to visit an old haunt or a place of interest, can lift your spirits and give you a sense of anticipation and excitement.

How to do it

It's best to start local and go farther afield when you feel more confident. You may wish to take along family or friends for company.

■ Visit places that may be comforting for people with dementia, such as small gardens that are easy to navigate, and movie theaters that show old films but eliminate lengthy trailers that could cause confusion.

■ Do not try to visit too many places in one outing.

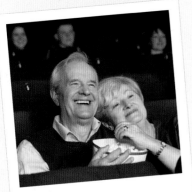
Movies

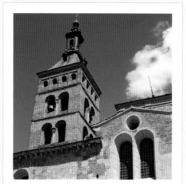
Local attraction

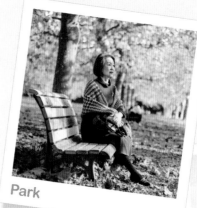
Park

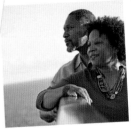
Short vacation

AT A GLANCE

✓ Active

✓ 1 or more people

✓ Productivity/leisure

✓ Variable timeframe

✓ Variable difficulty

! Identify potential risks, such as traffic, terrain, steps, crowds, or isolation

HOW IT HELPS

Going with a companion allows you to share experiences and create new memories together.

• A trip outdoors improves sleep, appetite, and vitamin D levels.

• Visiting old haunts can prompt episodic memories, such as street names in the area and the route you walked to school.

• Your new memories of your outing can spark conversation and improve your verbal expression as you recall them.

• Being out and about can help to reduce social isolation.

TALK ABOUT...

Places you might visit

• What were your favorite childhood outings?

• Favorite sweet treats for a journey

▲ Find out about places of interest using online websites, personal recommendations, or local tourist information offices.

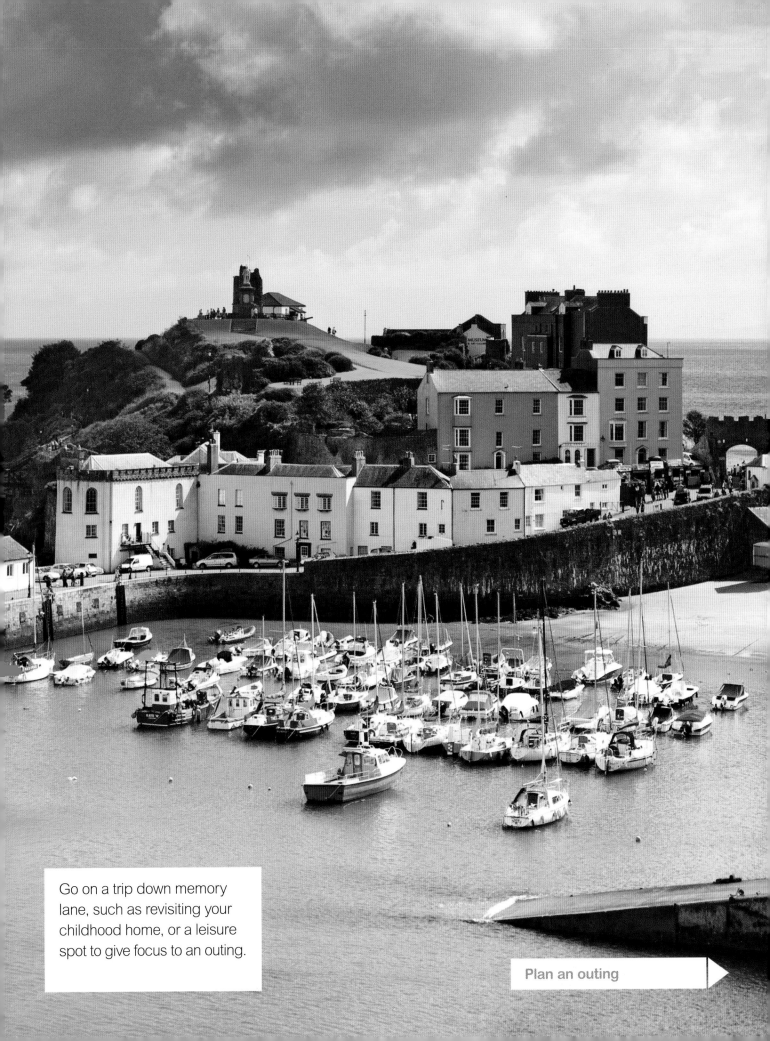

Go on a trip down memory lane, such as revisiting your childhood home, or a leisure spot to give focus to an outing.

Plan an outing ▶

Plan an outing

Planning your outing can be just as much fun as the outing itself, and it can help you minimize unnecessary stress on the day of your trip.

How to do it

You could enlist the help of family and friends in planning your outing.

■ Plan to travel at a time that suits you; "off-peak" times are usually quieter.

■ Consider whether it is realistic to go there and be back in a day: will you need to stay overnight?

■ If you are not feeling up to it on the day or if the weather is bad, postpone your trip for another day.

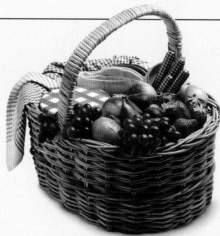

▲ Why not have a picnic at your local park or nature spot with friends or family?

HOW IT HELPS

Discussing plans with those around you maintains your communication skills and keeps you socially connected.

• Researching a trip involves a range of cognitive skills, including planning, organization, thinking, and reasoning.

• You use memory and orientation skills to plan routes and problem solving to assess the best travel option.

• Planning an outing can help you to feel in control of your choices, and improve your confidence and sense of self-worth.

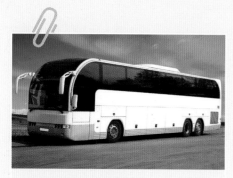

Transportation
A car will take you door to door, but you may prefer to use a bus, coach, or train, or go on an organized tour.

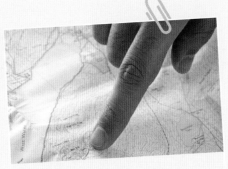

Distance
Consider how far the destination is from home. How will you get there and how long will it take you to travel?

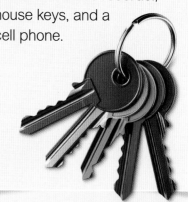

Essentials
Take everything you need— for example medication, a camera or video recorder, house keys, and a cell phone.

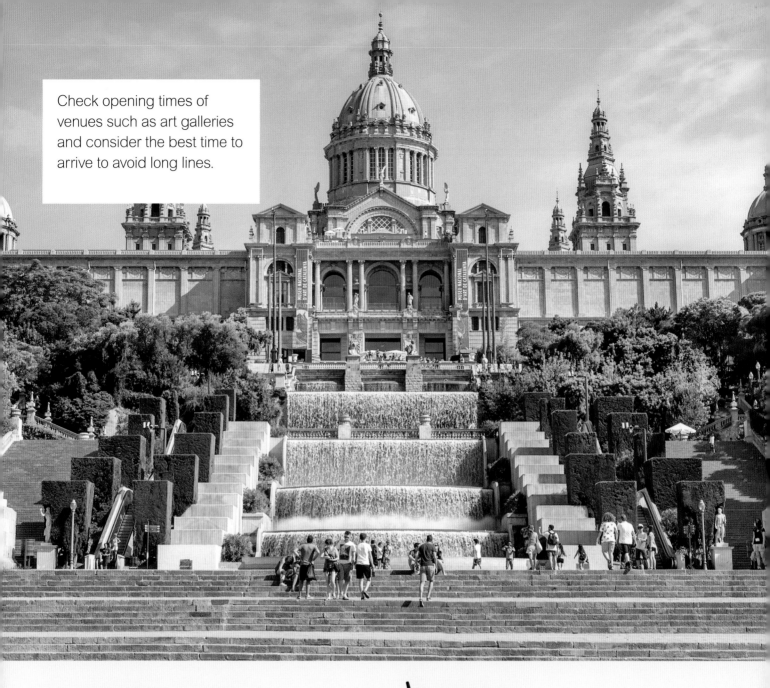

Check opening times of venues such as art galleries and consider the best time to arrive to avoid long lines.

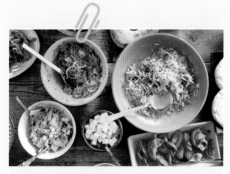

Plan a break
Build in regular pit stops to stretch your legs, use the toilet, have a drink and snack, or eat lunch.

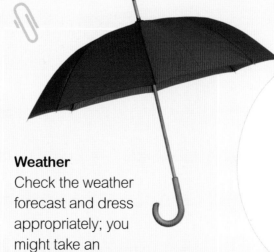

Weather
Check the weather forecast and dress appropriately; you might take an umbrella in case of rain.

You might want to take a camera or camcorder to capture memories of your outing

Make sure your cell phone has easily accessible emergency numbers

USEFUL TIPS

Get into the garden

Just being in the garden is good for you. You may have a green thumb and enjoy being busy in your garden, but simply sitting awhile or puttering around is also beneficial.

How to do it

There are jobs to be done year-round, so work at a comfortable pace and enjoy your garden.

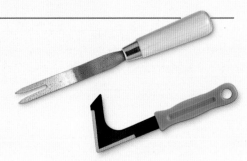

▲ Take care using sharp tools such as daisy grubbers or razor hoes.

■ Choose activities based on your skills and abilities. Sowing seeds of annuals is easy and gives rewarding results in a short time.

■ You may enjoy taking a trip to the local garden center or nursery or joining a local gardening group.

■ If mobility is a challenge, look through gardening books or watch your favorite gardening shows.

▶ Garden tasks can be relaxing as well as productive, and sharing tasks offers an opportunity to be sociable.

AT A GLANCE

✓ Active

✓ 1 or more persons

✓ Productivity

✓ No timeframe

✓ Variable difficulty

! Beware of trip hazards
! Exercise caution when handling tools and chemicals
! Avoid contact with poisonous and thorny plants

HOW IT HELPS

As well as the physical benefits of improved strength, mobility, and general fitness, gardening has recognized benefits for your mental health.

• The activity gives you a sense of purpose and achievement, which improves mood and well-being.

• Gardening utilizes your cognitive skills to plan, follow a sequence, concentrate, problem-solve, and remember.

• Being in the garden in all types of weather and seasons helps to orientate you to time.

• Stimulating all the senses outdoors can reduce anxiety and agitation.

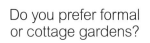
Watering

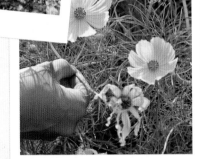
Deadheading

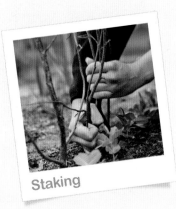
Staking

Do you prefer formal or cottage gardens?

•

Describe your favorite flower

•

Would you rather grow flowers or vegetables?

TALK ABOUT...

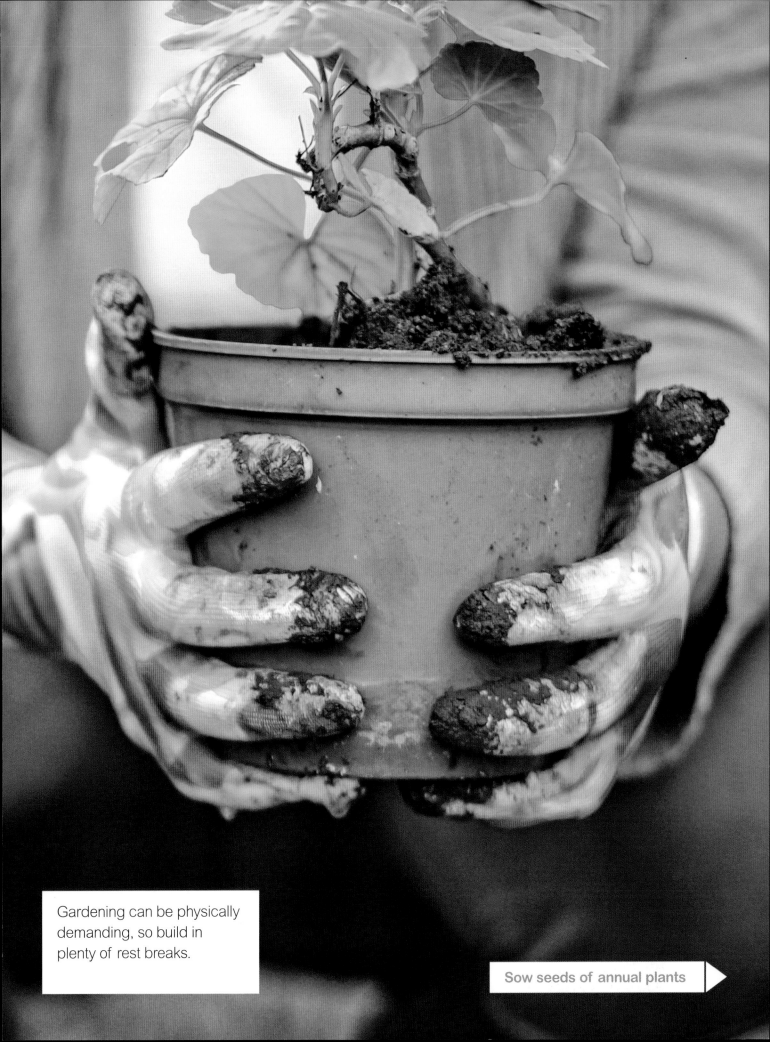

Gardening can be physically demanding, so build in plenty of rest breaks.

Sow seeds of annual plants ▷

Sow seeds of annual plants

Annuals flower earlier if you sow seeds indoors in early spring. Keep the pots in a greenhouse, cold frame, propagator, or on a windowsill to germinate the seeds. Then harden off the seedlings, to get them used to outdoor conditions, by putting them outside for a few hours each day.

WHAT YOU NEED
- 3½in (9cm) pots
- Trowel (optional)
- Potting soil
- Watering can with fine spray
- Packets of annual seeds
- Labels
- Perlite (if needed)
- Waterproof pen
- Propagator (optional)

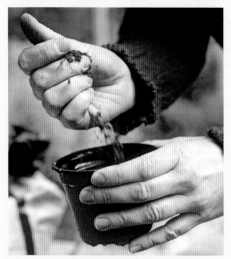

1 Fill each pot with soil, leaving a 1in (2.5cm) gap below the rim. Level the surface and press down gently.

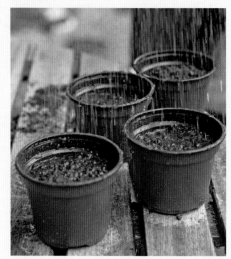

2 Once you have filled the pots, water using a watering can with a fine spray—it avoids disturbing the soil.

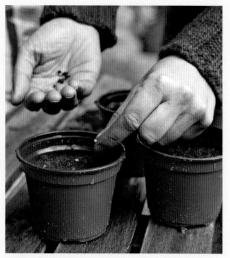

3 Plant small seeds evenly over the soil. For large seeds, like sunflower seeds, plant only 1 seed per pot.

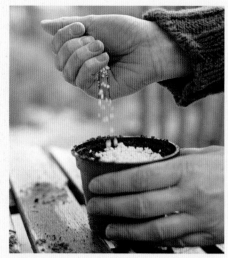

4 Cover the seeds with a layer of soil or, if they need light to germinate, some perlite. Check the seed packet.

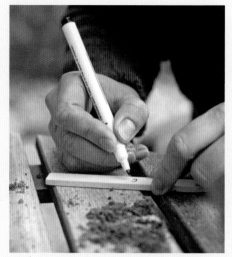

5 Label each pot with the name of the plant and date. Leave in a bright place out of direct sun to germinate.

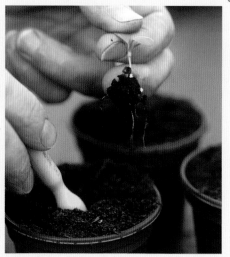

6 Thin seedlings to leave the sturdiest one in each pot or replant them in individual pots of fresh soil.

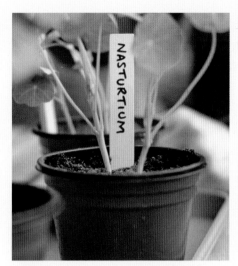

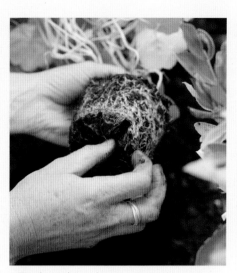

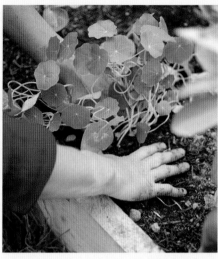

7 Once the seedlings have 2–4 pairs of true leaves, move the pots outdoors each day for two weeks to harden them off.

8 Let the plants grow in pots until big enough to be planted. Knock each one out of its pot and tease out its roots.

9 Put it in the planting hole, which should be a little wider than and as deep as the rootball. Fill in the hole and press gently.

▼ Many annual plants look great in hanging baskets and other containers, as well as borders.

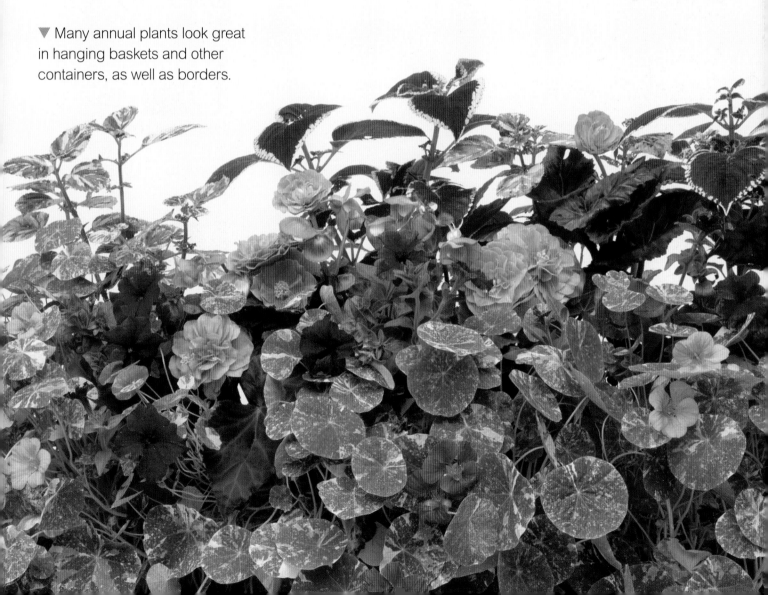

Create a sensory garden

It is healthy to stimulate your senses and you can easily do so by enhancing any outside space, large or small, with sensory objects.

How to do it

Do as much as your available space, budget, and gardening skills allow. Think of ways you can adapt the ideas shown here.

■ Use varying textures of wood, stone, and bark in the paving, fencing or trellis, seats and containers, and ornaments.

■ Fountains or cascades that allow water to run safely through your fingers offer good stimulation for sight, hearing, and touch.

■ For extra visual stimulation, hang old CDs from branches.

■ A garden path leading in a circle is ideal. But make sure that it is easy to navigate and is of the same material and color.

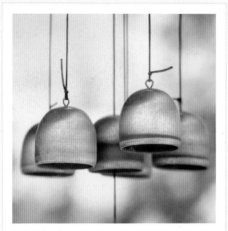

Wind chimes

▲ Add features such as wind chimes for sound, a fountain to touch and listen to, and a windcatcher to attract the eye.

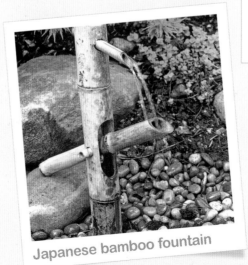

Japanese bamboo fountain

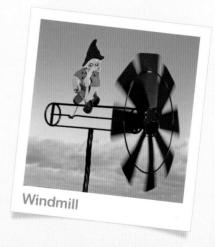

Windmill

AT A GLANCE

✓ Active

✓ 1 or more people

✓ Productivity

✓ No timeframe

✓ Variable difficulty

! Beware of trip hazards and be safe when handling tools and chemicals

! Avoid poisonous and thorny plants

HOW IT HELPS

Sensory gardens encourage you to venture outdoors and be aware of your environment.

• Stimulating the senses can trigger emotional memories and encourage reminiscence.

• Planning and creating a sensory garden employs cognitive skills such as reasoning, planning, problem-solving, ability to anticipate, and spatial awareness.

• Sensory gardens encourage you to relax, promoting mindfulness and alleviating restlessness and agitation.

• Your physical health also benefits from the reduction in stress and lowered blood pressure.

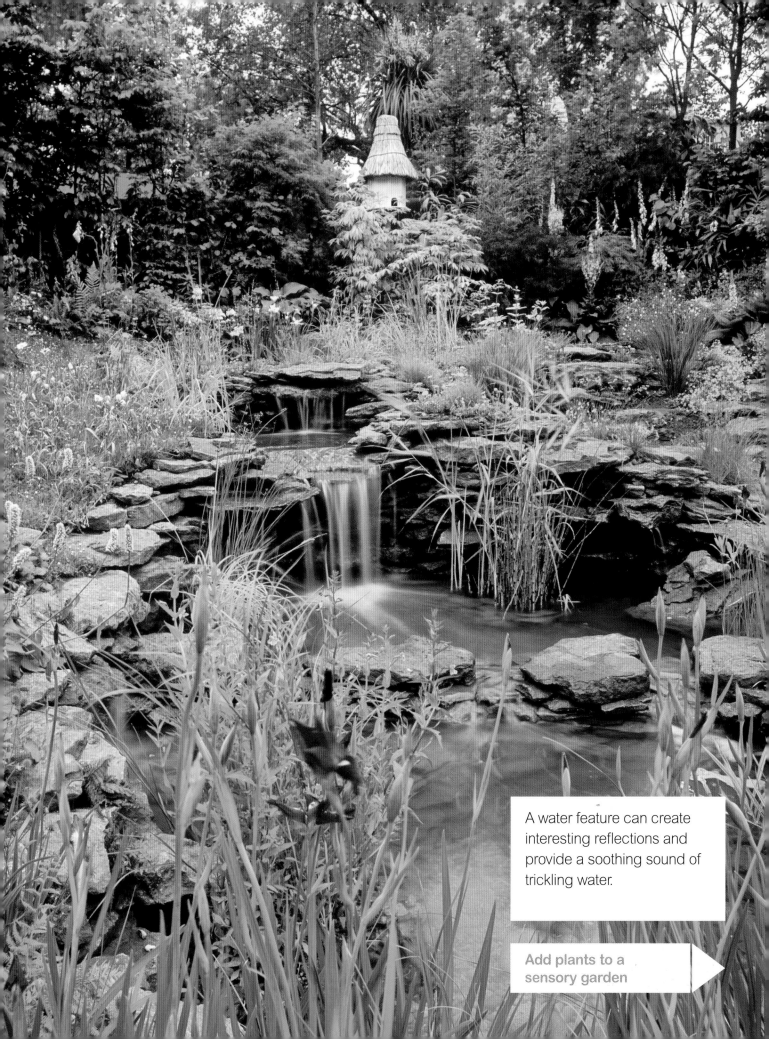

A water feature can create interesting reflections and provide a soothing sound of trickling water.

Add plants to a
sensory garden

Add plants to a sensory garden

Enhance the sensory experience of your garden by choosing plants that stimulate all five senses.

How to do it

A few suitable plants are listed in the planting ideas box below, but there are many more to choose from.

■ Contrast plants that are soft to touch with other textures, such as smooth stones.

■ Look for ideas in books or online (or talk to a friend) to find plants that you like and that are easy to grow.

■ Visiting a nursery or public garden can make it easier to choose the best plants.

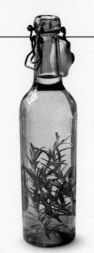

▲ Use herbs from the garden to flavor olive oil or to intensify flavors in your cooking.

AT A GLANCE

✓ Active or sedentary

✓ 1 or more people

✓ Productivity

✓ No timeframe

✓ Variable difficulty

❗ Beware of trip hazards and be safe when handling tools and chemicals

❗ Avoid poisonous and thorny plants

HOW IT HELPS

Seeing, touching, feeling, smelling, and tasting the plants around you can stimulate memories and conversations.

• Enjoying sensory plants with a family member or friend helps your social interaction skills.

• Making your own choice of plants helps to maintain your sense of self-worth, value, and self-esteem.

PLANTING IDEAS

• Sight: heucheras, marigolds, palms, rhubarb
• Sound: greater quaking grass, sweetcorn
• Touch: California poppies, lamb's ears, silver sage
• Smell: curry plant, jasmine, lilies, rosemary, roses
• Taste: basil, chives, mint, raspberries, tomatoes

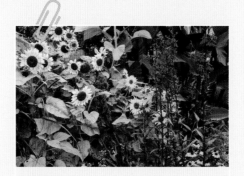

Sight
Use plants with varying heights and forms, colorful flowers, and leaves with contrasting sizes and shapes.

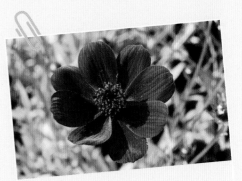

Smell
Some plants have fragrant leaves or flowers, like this chocolate cosmos: plant near a seat, path, or pergola.

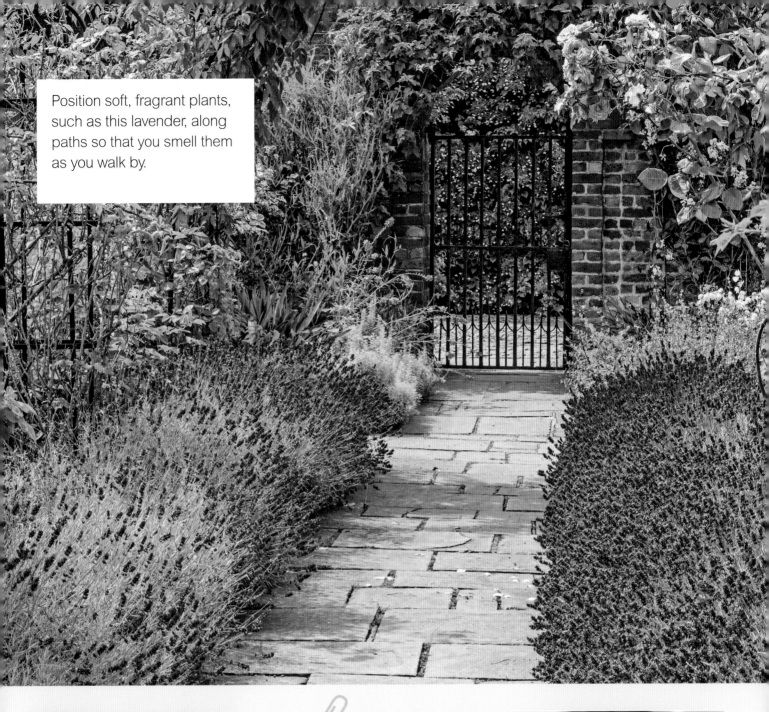

Position soft, fragrant plants, such as this lavender, along paths so that you smell them as you walk by.

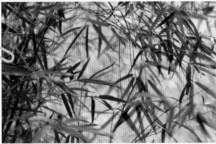

Sound
Perennial bamboos and grasses have papery leaves that rustle in the breeze.

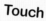

Touch
Some plants have silky petals or velvety leaves, and grasses may have soft flower heads.

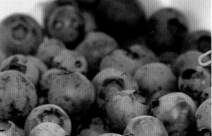

Taste
There are lots of edible plants to pick and enjoy: try herbs or soft fruits like blueberries.

Plant a container

Containers are easy to plant and maintain, and watching the plants grow will give you a great sense of achievement.

Making the task easier

Gather together everything you need in advance: plants, soil, and tools. Choose a frost-proof container with plenty of drainage holes.

■ Work at waist height to minimize any bending and stretching. You could work sitting at a table if you prefer.

▲ Gardening tools with good, solid or long handles may be more comfortable to use.

■ Consider the weight of the planted container— you may need help to lift it into position or you could plant it in situ.

■ If your visual perception is not good, choose a container and plants with bright, contrasting colors to help you to distinguish shapes.

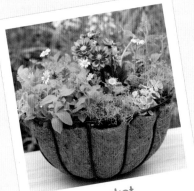

Hanging basket

HOW IT HELPS

Planting a container with friends or family gives you the opportunity to make it a social activity, and a chance to catch up and reminisce.

• Involves sensory elements such as feeling the soil, smelling the plants, and looking at the flowers, which can stimulate episodic memories and have a calming feeling.

• Uses a range of cognitive skills, in planning and arranging the plants, problem-solving and concentration, as well as initiating, sequencing, and completing a task.

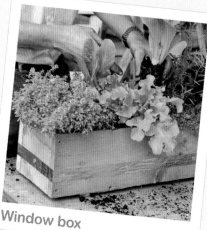

Window box

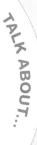

Favorite type of container

•

Growing flowers or growing vegetables?

•

Good plants to grow in window boxes

TALK ABOUT...

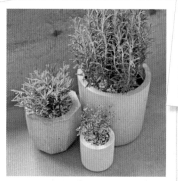

Patio containers

◀ As well as window boxes, plant containers for the balcony, patio, or to mark paths through the garden.

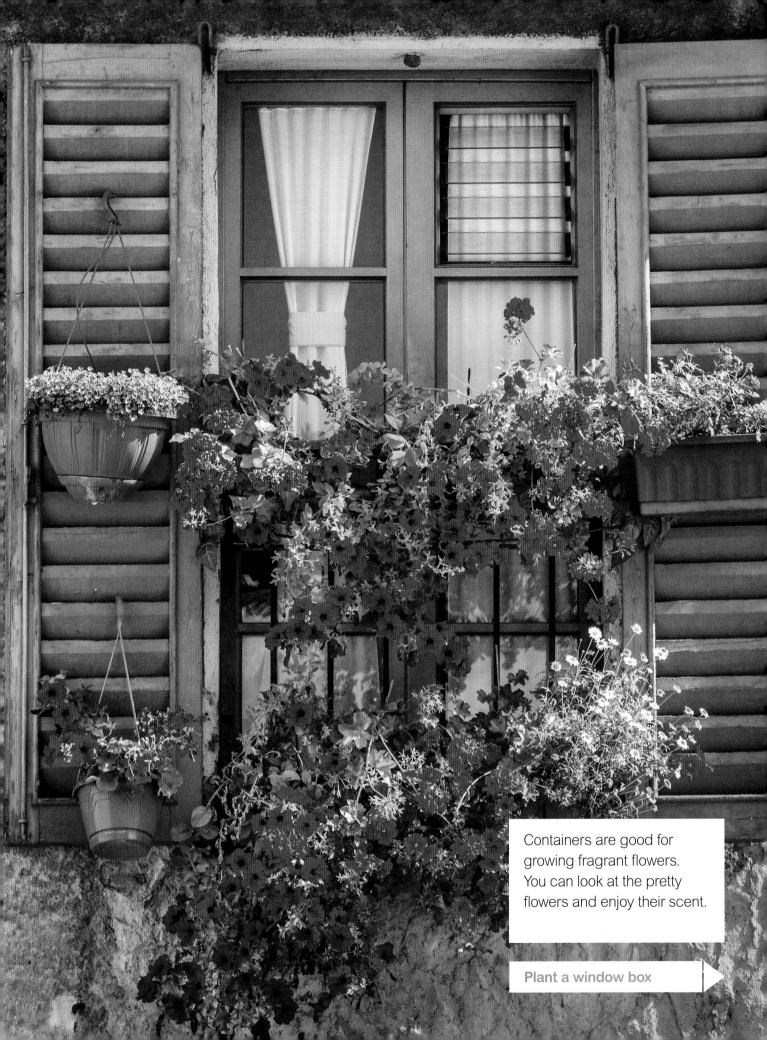

Containers are good for growing fragrant flowers. You can look at the pretty flowers and enjoy their scent.

Plant a window box ▶

Plant a window box

The plants in this window box provide beautiful scents from the foliage and pretty flowers, as well as tasty herbs for you to pick from summer to early fall. You could use different plants, if you prefer. If you are comfortable with woodworking, you could also make a window box at home (see pages 176–179).

WHAT YOU NEED

- All-purpose general fertilizer
- Multipurpose potting soil
- Packing peanuts
- Trowel
- Window box, about 18 x 8 x 8 in (45 x 20 x 20 cm)
- 2 scented-leaved geraniums, such as "Orange Fizz" and "Attar of Roses"
- 1 red-veined sorrel (Rumex sanguineus)
- 1 creeping thyme (Thymus serpyllum)
- 1 variegated oregano (Origanum vulgare "Country Cream")
- 1 Thai basil (Ocimum basilicum var. thyrsiflorum)
- Watering can

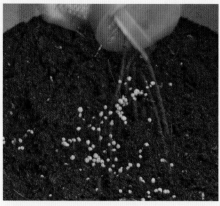

1 Mix some fertilizer into the soil (add some at the rate recommended by the manufacturer).

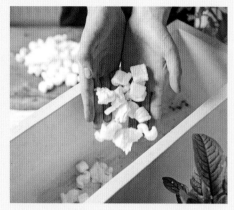

2 To prevent the holes from clogging with soil, put a thin layer of packing peanuts over the base of the box.

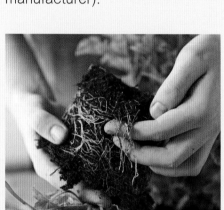

6 Knock the plant out of its pot. Gently work the roots to release them and encourage them to grow out.

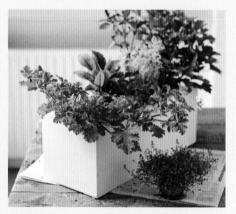

7 Sit the plant back on the soil and add more plants, checking that each is set 1 in (2.5 cm) below the rim.

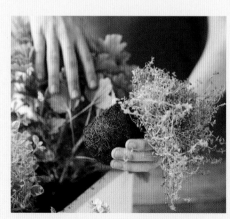

9 Tuck in the low, creeping plants, such as the thyme, at the front, where they will not be overshadowed.

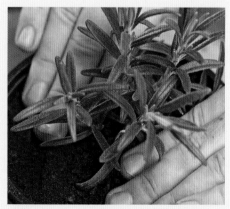

10 When the window box is full, fill in any gaps with soil and press gently around all the rootballs.

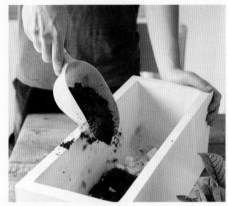

3 Add at least 2 in (5 cm) of soil so that the packing peanuts are completely covered.

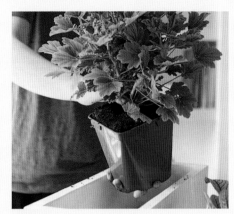

4 Put the largest plant in its pot in the center. Check that the top of the root ball sits about 1 in (2.5 cm) below the rim.

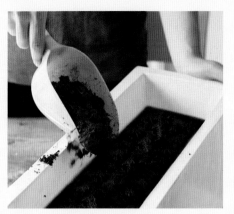

5 If the pot is too high or too low, take out or add soil and try the pot again until it is at the correct level.

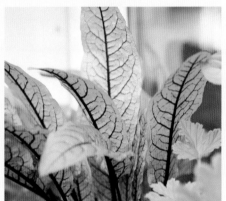

8 Put the taller-growing plants, like this sorrel, toward the back of the window box.

▼ As well as using the herb leaves in cooking, you could use the thyme flowers to decorate salads.

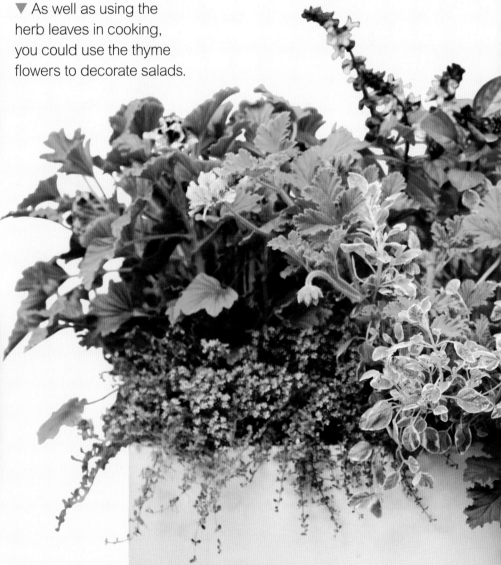

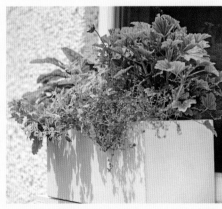

11 Set the window box on a windowsill and water well to settle the soil. Make sure the box is sitting securely.

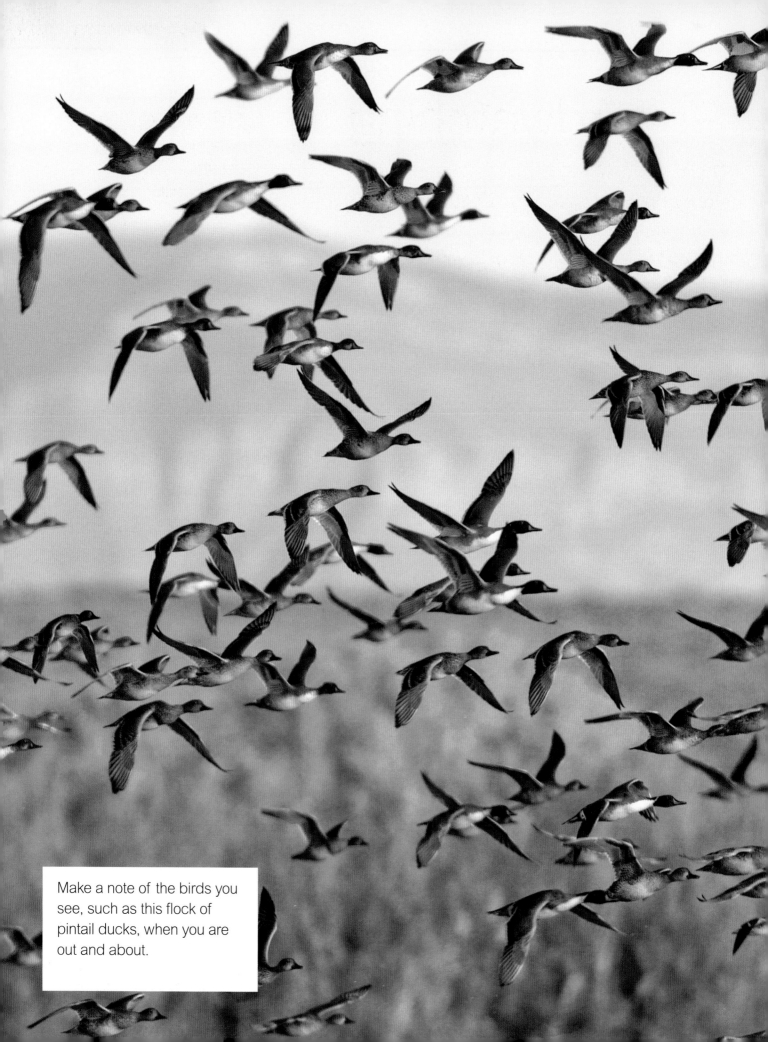

Make a note of the birds you see, such as this flock of pintail ducks, when you are out and about.

Go birdwatching

There is a simple joy to be derived from the sight and sounds of birds. Go outdoors to watch them or position your armchair by the window so you can see them from the comfort of your living room.

HOW IT HELPS

Listening to birdsong is proven to help people to relax.

• By stimulating the senses, listening to birdsong reduces agitation.

• Recording bird activity utilizes cognitive skills such as thinking, recognition, and organization, as well as memory recall.

How to do it

Encourage birds into your garden with bird feeders and tables, bird baths, nesting boxes, and plants with berries and seeds.

■ Go outside to listen to the dawn chorus—it can be an uplifting experience. If this is not practical, buy a recording of birdsong.

■ Write in a notebook or nature diary about any bird activity you see.

■ Join a local or national birdwatching organization to share your interest with fellow enthusiasts.

■ Consult reference books or the internet to find out more about the species you have seen.

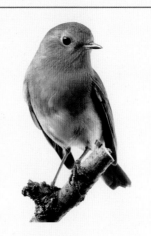

▲ If you notice some birds that are regular garden visitors, you could take part in a local or national count of bird numbers in your area.

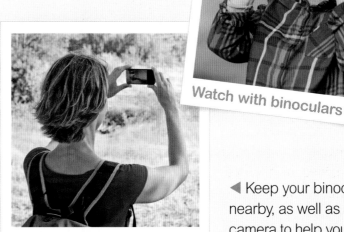

Watch with binoculars

Take photographs

◀ Keep your binoculars nearby, as well as a camera to help you identify unfamiliar species later.

TALK ABOUT...

Talking birds

•

Do you like common birds or exotic birds?

•

Can you mimic birdsong?

•

What is a common name for a "birdwatcher?"

Feed the birds

Encourage birds to come into your garden by putting out a range of tasty treats. You could even make your own bird food.

How to do it

Establish a routine for tending birds that includes feeding, providing fresh water, and keeping feeders clean.

■ Consider using prompts to remind you to feed the birds: make a memory card (see pages 204–207) or put an alert on your cell phone.

■ You can put leftovers, such as fruit, stale cheese, potato, and cooked rice, on a bird table.

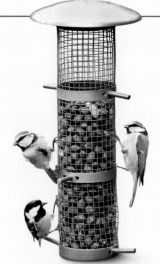

▲ An easy option is to use one of the many ready-made bird feeders available.

▶ There are many types of bird food and feeders: put out a variety to entice different birds.

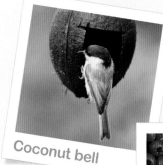

Coconut bell

HOW IT HELPS

Taking responsibility for the regular task of feeding the birds can enhance your self-worth.

• A daily routine gives a natural rhythm to the day, helping you to remain orientated to time.

• Making bird food involves a range of cognitive skills such as planning, organization, following sequences and completing a task, and concentration.

• Stringing fruit and nuts for a bird-food streamer requires good hand-eye coordination and fine finger movement.

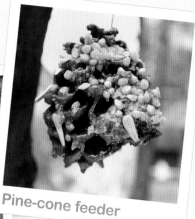

Pine-cone feeder

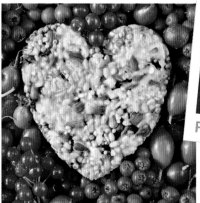

Cookie-cutter suet cake

TALK ABOUT...

What birds do you see in your garden?

•

City squares often have pigeons—are they pretty or pests?

•

Did you know that throwing bread to ducks is bad for them?

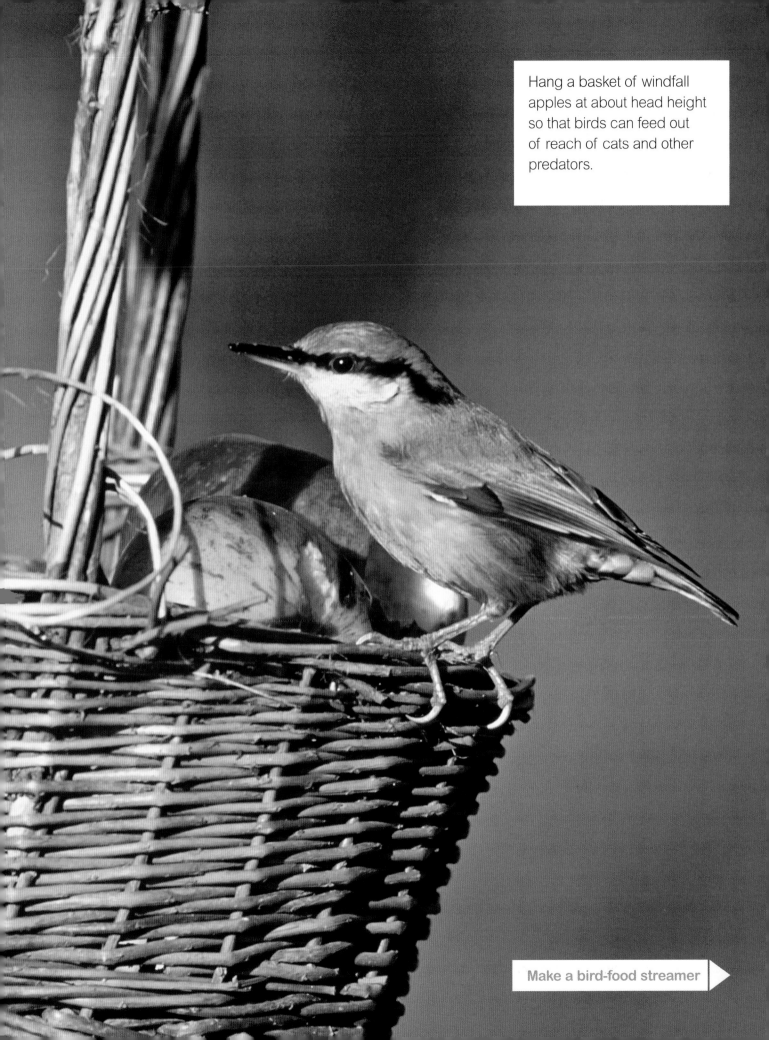

Hang a basket of windfall apples at about head height so that birds can feed out of reach of cats and other predators.

Make a bird-food streamer ▷

Make a bird-food streamer

This bird-food streamer is easy and fun to make, especially if you prepare it with friends or family. Gather your ingredients together first. If you are unsure of any part of the preparation, such as slicing the apples, concentrate on the parts you feel confident with, and get someone else to help.

WHAT YOU NEED

- 2 or 3 large pine cones
- Natural-fiber, soft garden twine
- Scissors
- Butter knife
- Peanut butter
- Good quality wild bird seed (it should not contain split peas, lentils, or dried rice)
- Peanuts (in the shell)
- Dried fruit
- Large-eyed needle
- Apples
- Apple corer
- Kitchen knife
- Chopping board
- Piece of raffia

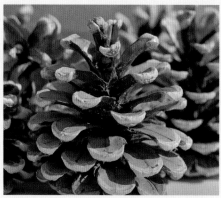

1 Choose pine cones with fully open, spreading scales. Tie a length of twine securely to the top of each cone.

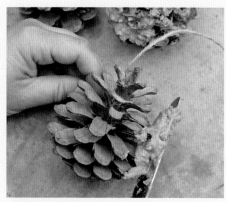

2 Take the butter knife and use it to smear peanut butter all over each pine cone, pushing it into all the gaps.

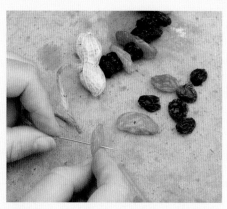

6 Thread the needle with a piece of twine and knot the end. Use the needle to thread nuts and fruit on the twine.

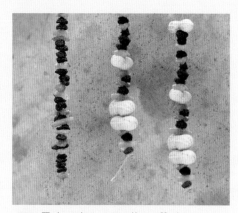

7 Take the needle off the twine and repeat step 6 to make more bird-food chains.

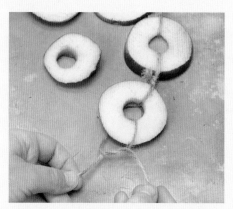

9 Tie about five of the apple rings together with loops of string into a chain. Leave some extra twine at the top.

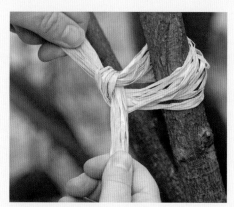

10 Take the raffia into the garden. Tie it securely between two sturdy branches at eye level, pulling it taut.

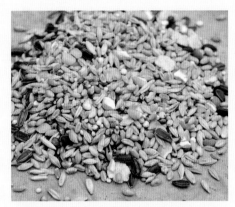

3 Spread a few handfuls of the seed mix in a heap over your work surface.

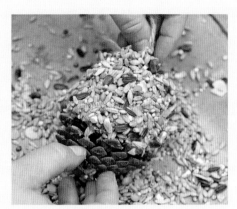

4 Roll each cone in the seed mix until the peanut butter is completely covered. Press in more seed with your fingers.

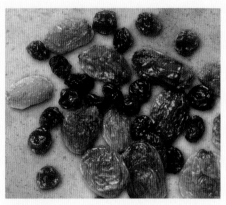

5 Next, get the peanuts and dried fruit ready to make a bird-food chain. Discard any moldy nuts.

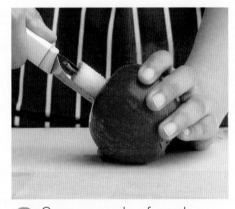

8 Core a couple of apples. Use the kitchen knife to slice the apples on a chopping board to make apple rings.

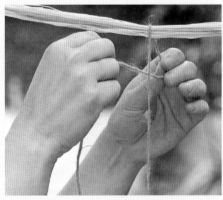

11 Tie the pine cones, bird-food chains, and apple rings to the raffia. Then wait for the birds to come.

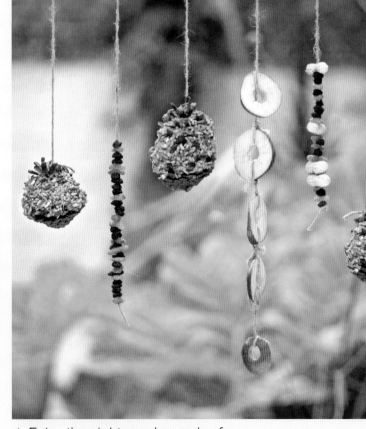

▲ Enjoy the sights and sounds of birds coming into your garden to feed on the bird-food streamer that you have put together.

Indoor gardening

If you do not have a garden or find it difficult to get around outdoors, bring the garden indoors. You can still enjoy activities such as growing potted plants indoors and on a windowsill.

How to do it

Grow plants that you like, but choose ones that will thrive indoors. Try ornamental plants, such as begonia or ivy, and edible plants such as herbs or easy vegetables.

■ When preparing to plant or to sow indoors, first prepare everything you will need, such as soil, tools, and plants.

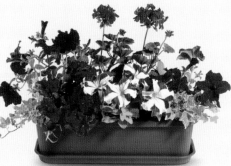

▲ Don't forget the windowsill—it's just the place for a window box.

▶ Here are a few suggestions for easy plants to grow indoors, but also look online or in gardening books for more ideas.

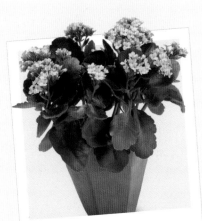

Flaming Katy

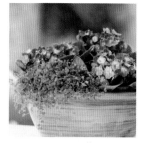

African violets

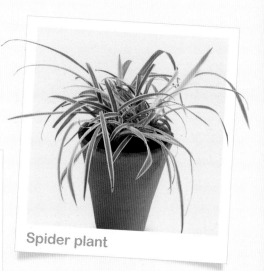

Spider plant

AT A GLANCE

✓ Gentle activity

✓ 1 person

✓ Productivity

✓ 20 minutes

✓ Simple

! Involves use of scissors

HOW IT HELPS

Indoor gardening can improve the air quality of your home and enhance your well-being.

• Growing plants indoors stimulates the senses with color and fragrance, as well as taste if you include herbs or vegetables.

• Incorporating raw and healthy foods into your diet provides extra vitamins and minerals, which benefit your health.

• You utilize a range of physical skills to handle the plants and manipulate tools.

• Cognitive skills, particularly concentration and attention, are needed to complete the activity.

TALK ABOUT...

Other plants you could grow indoors

What is a terrarium?

Herbs that you enjoy growing and eating

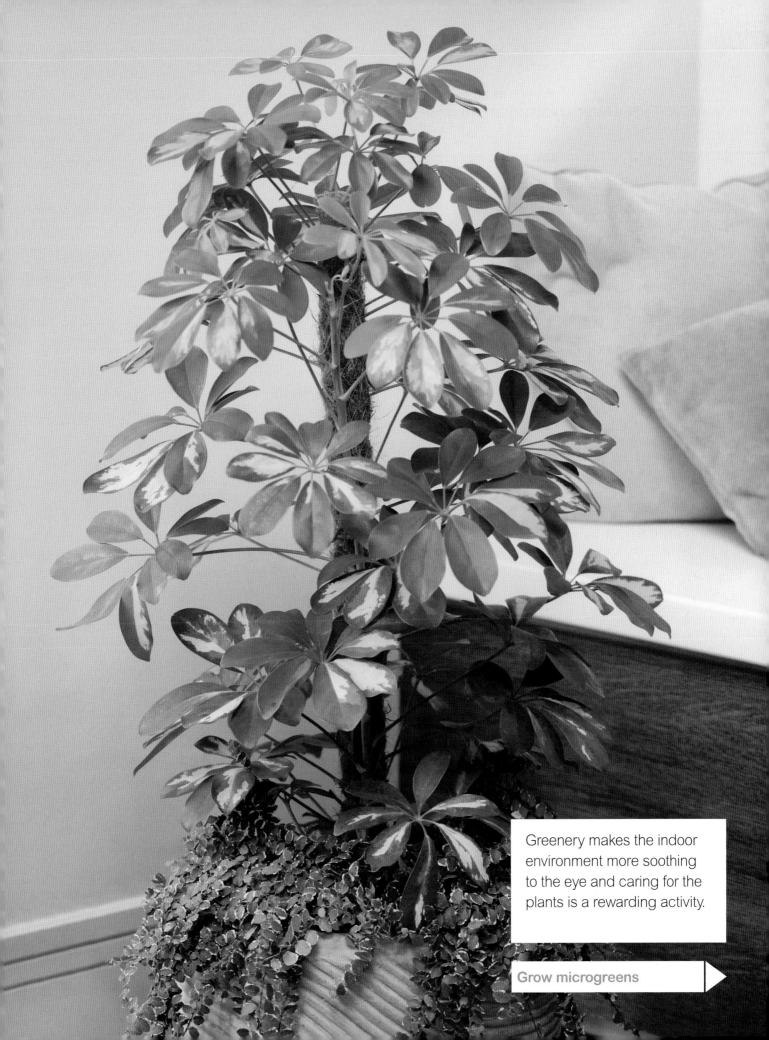

Greenery makes the indoor environment more soothing to the eye and caring for the plants is a rewarding activity.

Grow microgreens ▶

Grow microgreens in muffin cups

Microgreens are the leaves of lettuces, herbs, or peas that are harvested when still tiny. They are great in salads or as a garnish and may be up to 40 percent more nutritious than bigger plants. Microgreens are ready to eat in about 10 days.

WHAT YOU NEED

- Microgreens seed mix
- Bowl of water
- Large silicone muffin cups
- Scissors
- Potting soil
- Vermiculite
- Waterproof tray
- Watering can
- Pocket snips
  or kitchen scissors

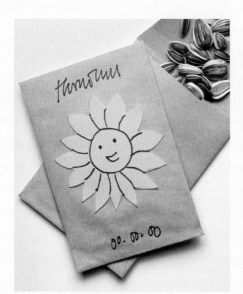

1 Soak large seeds, such as sunflower seeds, overnight in a bowl of water before sowing, to help them to germinate.

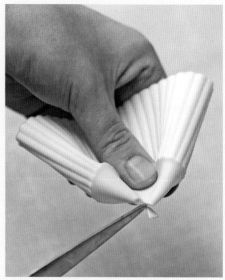

2 Fold the muffin cup in half. With sharp scissors, snip off the bottom to create a small drainage hole.

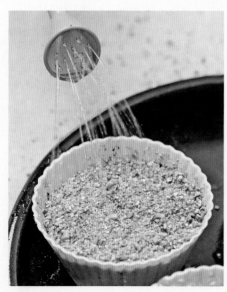

6 Put the muffin cup on a tray and water it gently. Place the tray on a bright windowsill out of direct sun.

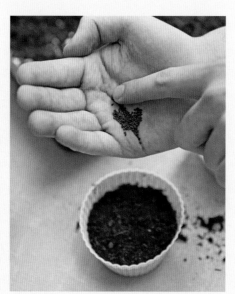

7 Sow one cup every few days for a continuous crop of microgreens that can be harvested over a longer period.

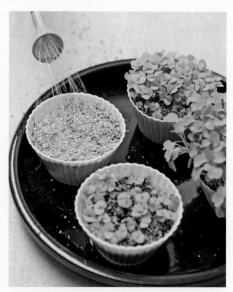

8 Water the plants and turn the cups regularly. Turning the cups will ensure that the stems grow straight.

Other containers

You can use other containers such as plant pots, egg cartons, or yogurt cups. Wash them first and cut a drainage hole in each bottom.

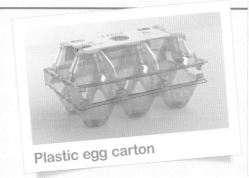
Plastic egg carton

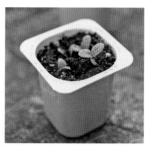
Yogurt cup

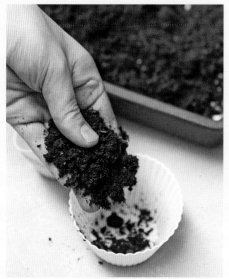

3 Fill the cup with soil, leaving a ¼ in (5 mm) gap at the top. Press the soil gently with your fingers.

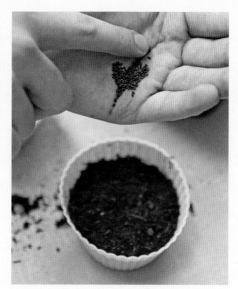

4 Sow the seeds thickly and evenly over the soil. Lightly press them into the surface with your fingertips.

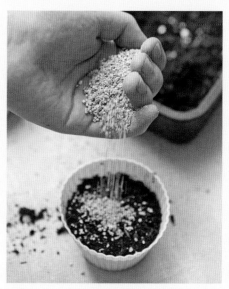

5 Cover the seeds with a thin layer of vermiculite to keep the seeds moist and let in some light, so they germinate well.

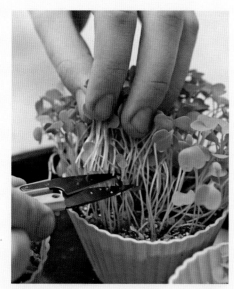

9 Once the first true leaves have grown, use pocket snips or scissors to cut the shoots as needed.

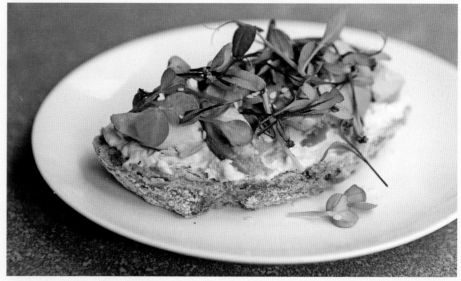

▲ Enjoy freshly harvested microgreens on a sandwich, in a salad, or as a tasty garnish to a hot dish.

REVISITING THE PAST

Reminiscing is a great activity because it triggers memories of events in your life and of how you felt about them. Some memories may be positive, others not so good—enjoy focusing on the moments that make you happy and proud. Talking about your life with family and friends can make you feel more connected to them and boost your spirits. Explore the many ways to revisit your past to recapture the thoughts, feelings, and memories that shaped your life.

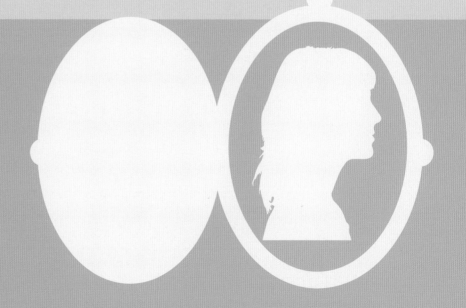

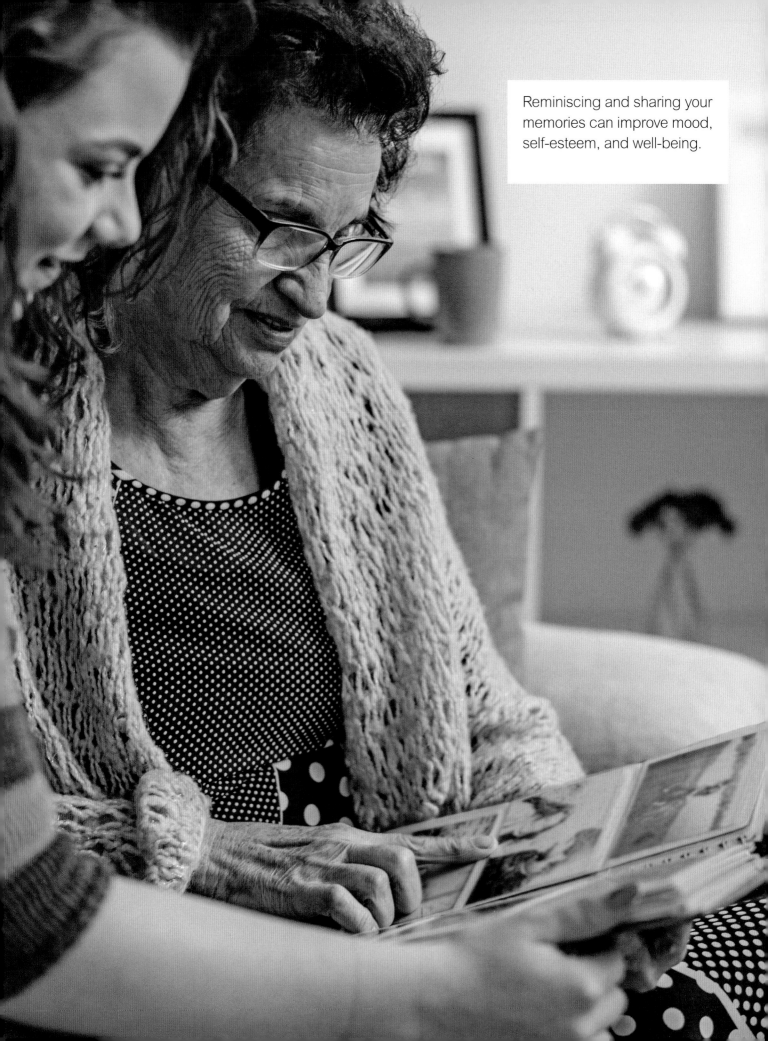

Reminiscing and sharing your memories can improve mood, self-esteem, and well-being.

Bring out the photos

If you can remember your early life better than recent events, try looking at old photos of family events, your home town, or places you have visited. These photos can trigger memories that you could share with family and friends.

How to do it

You are the expert on the events of your life so this is a failure-free activity.

■ Get larger copies of photos if needed, so that they are easier to see and to protect the originals.

■ It is helpful if photos are marked with details such as who is in them, where it is, and the date. Ask someone to help you if you are struggling to remember the details.

■ As you look at and handle the photos, recount the stories and memories that they trigger.

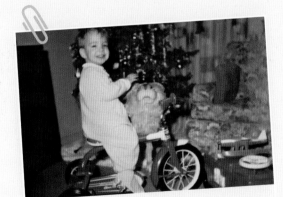

Meaningful memories
Limit the number of photographs that you look at each time; one image may be enough to enjoy.

HOW IT HELPS

Looking at and holding old photos can be a good conversation starter, using your communication skills and keeping you socially engaged.

• Photos can stimulate emotional memories—of how you felt at the time the photograph was taken.

• Recalling events, people, and places improves cognition skills and facial recognition, helping you to stay orientated.

• Remembering the past can sometimes unlock forgotten skills—for instance, looking at an old school photo may help you to remember historical dates or a poem that you learned at school.

When did you get your first camera?

•

Black-and-white versus color photos

•

Past fashions: trendy or fashion faux pas?

•

Film versus digital photos

TALK ABOUT...

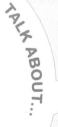

Compile a photo album

If you organize your photos into one or more albums, you can create a lasting record for you to enjoy and share with others.

How to do it

Before you start sorting your photos, decide on a theme to help you choose. You might decide to make more than one album.

■ Try using an online company to create an album from your digital photos. Ask for help if you haven't done it before.

■ If you sort the photos on a tray, you can put them away easily if you want to take a break and finish later.

▲ You could make smaller albums with photos of your pets.

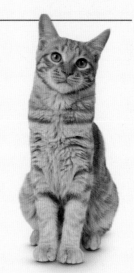

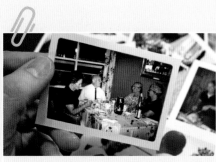

Sort your photos
Gather and sort your photos before putting them in the album. Pick your favorites and arrange them in order.

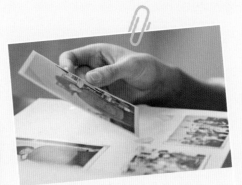

A suitable album
Albums with plastic pockets or self-adhesive pages to hold your photos are easy to use.

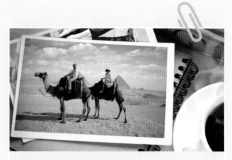

Choosing a theme
Your album could be a record of your life, a memorable event such as a vacation, or a hobby or passion.

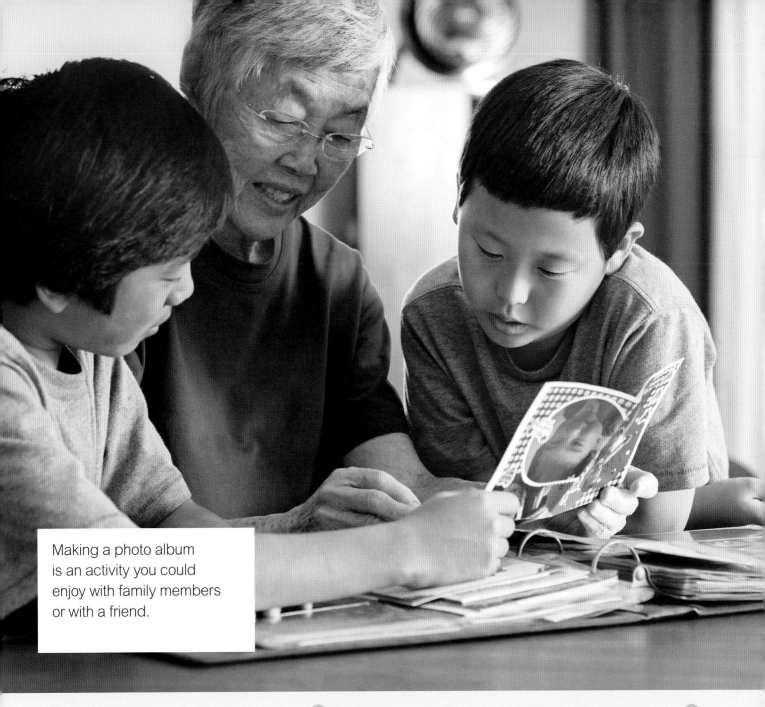

Making a photo album is an activity you could enjoy with family members or with a friend.

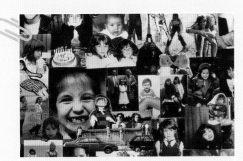

Photo collage
You could display a few of your favorite photos in frames or use them to create a collage.

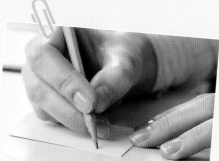

Labeling
Label each photo with the occasion, names of people and the place, and date.

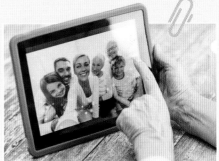

Digital photo frame
Instead of filling a photo album, load your digital photos onto a digital photo frame.

Draw a family tree

Capture your family history to pass on to younger generations. It could be a one-off activity or a research project that sparks your imagination and starts a journey of discovery of long-lost family.

How to do it

Start by collecting all the information you need to draw a family tree. Make a note of what you already know and involve family members to fill in the gaps.

■ Use online genealogy websites or look at old records in local libraries and churches to help with your research. You might want to take someone with you to help take notes.

■ Use the template shown here to map out the information you need to put on the family tree.

■ Decide how you want to depict the family tree. You could draw your own tree, with family members spread along the branches, use a printed chart, or make a collage.

TALK ABOUT...

How many generations are there after you?

•

How many generations of your family can you recall?

•

Did you have a favorite relative?

•

How have lives changed over the span of your family tree?

HOW IT HELPS

Researching your family tree and sharing the results provides an opportunity to connect (or reconnect) with family members.

• The research calls on long-term, episodic memories, which are often more reliable than short-term memories, so it helps you to feel positive about your own abilities.

• The activity offers a good topic of conversation, promoting positive communication.

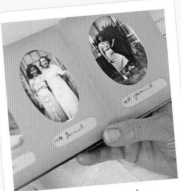

Family photographs

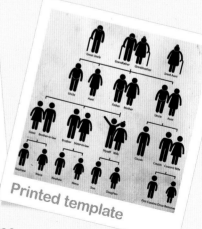

Printed template

▲ There are printed family tree templates available to fill in. You can add photographs to further personalize your family tree.

Use this simple template

Copy this template on to a large sheet of paper. Start by putting in your details first, in the center.

■ Add other members of your family as indicated. If you need to add more people, for example more siblings, draw some extra boxes.

■ Draw lines to connect the boxes—if people are divorced, draw a dotted line.

■ Put siblings on the same line, with the oldest to the left and youngest to the right.

■ You may want to add details such as dates of birth, marriages, and deaths.

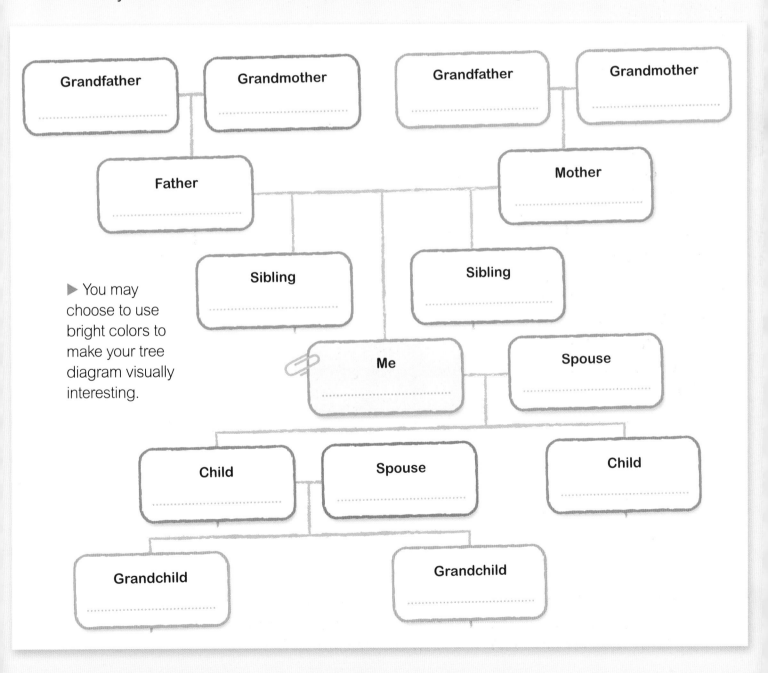

▶ You may choose to use bright colors to make your tree diagram visually interesting.

Fill a memory box

Each memory box will be unique and personal to you. Enjoy the process of filling it—and then of looking through it—on your own or use it to share memories with family and friends.

How to do it

Gather together your treasured keepsakes, then sort through them to pick out items suitable for a memory box.

■ Consider making labels or short story cards for the items to capture special memories.

■ Place the items in the box so that you can take them out whenever you want to revisit your memories.

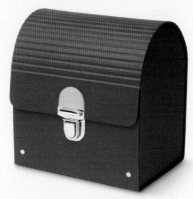

▲ Choose a sturdy box with a lid of a suitable size, such as a shoebox, jewelry box, or plastic storage box.

USEFUL TIPS

You might also include trophies, medals, knickknacks with sentimental value, or old photographs

•

Newspaper clippings can mark important dates

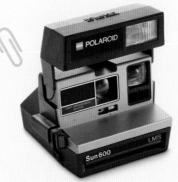

Hobbies
You could concentrate on objects of particular interest in your life, such as special items from a hobby collection.

AT A GLANCE

✓ Sedentary

✓ 1 or more people

✓ Productivity

✓ No time limit

✓ Easy

! May trigger negative as well as positive emotions

! Avoid heavy or sharp objects

HOW IT HELPS

The experience of handling physical objects benefits well-being in several ways.

• Seeing, smelling, and touching are all involved in processing information in the brain. They can help trigger long-term memories and benefit short-term memory.

• Sharing memories with others improves your communication skills and reinforces a sense of self by acknowledging your achievements in life.

• Keeping connected with those around you can enhance general mood and confidence.

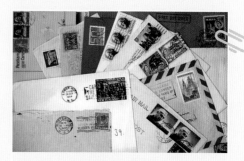

Correspondence
You may want to look through old letters a few at a time. They can stir up strong emotions.

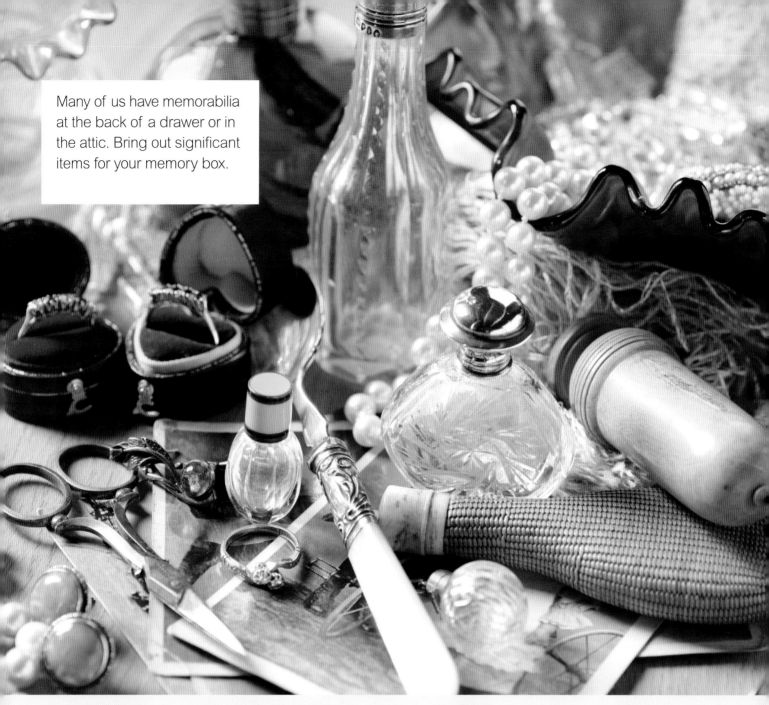

Many of us have memorabilia at the back of a drawer or in the attic. Bring out significant items for your memory box.

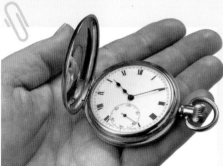

Family heirlooms
Include mementos from your life that are especially dear to you, such as family jewelry.

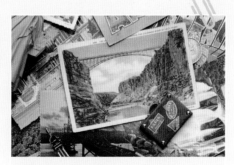

Themed boxes
Create boxes with different themes, such as a favorite band, sports team, or travels.

Lifetime stages
You may want memory boxes for different periods of your life, with an old toy or item of clothing in a childhood box, or business cards or name tags in a work-life box.

Fill a scrapbook

Scrapbooking is a popular way of displaying your passions and pastimes in a book. It can be as basic or as elaborate as you like.

How to do it

Gather everything you want to put in the scrapbook, as well as labels or paper on which to write memories, glue, scissors, and any decorations.

■ Use a red or contrasting tablecloth on your work surface to make items appear more distinct.

■ Do not overcrowd your workspace; you may find it distracting. Work on the scrapbook a little at a time.

■ Arrange one item on each page, along with any decorations. Write any labels or notes and attach them.

HOW IT HELPS

Filling a scrapbook lets you express your creativity and engenders a sense of accomplishment.

• This activity elicits episodic and emotional memories that can be recaptured when looking at the scrapbook.

• Practicing cognitive skills, such as planning, concentration, initiating, following sequences, task completion, and decision-making, may help the brain to retain them.

• Using a scrapbook to share stories with others aids your communication skills and keeps you connected to other people.

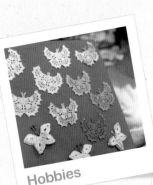
Hobbies

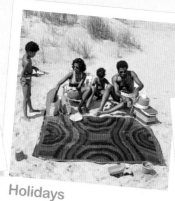
Holidays

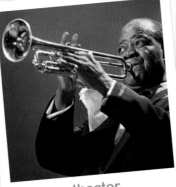
Music or theater

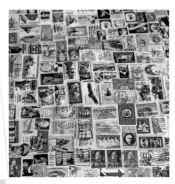
Collections

TALK ABOUT...

Favorite hobbies

Achievements relating to your hobby

Do you enjoy collecting?

Memorable events in your life

▲ Decide what theme you want for your scrapbook: it could be any subject or event that interests you.

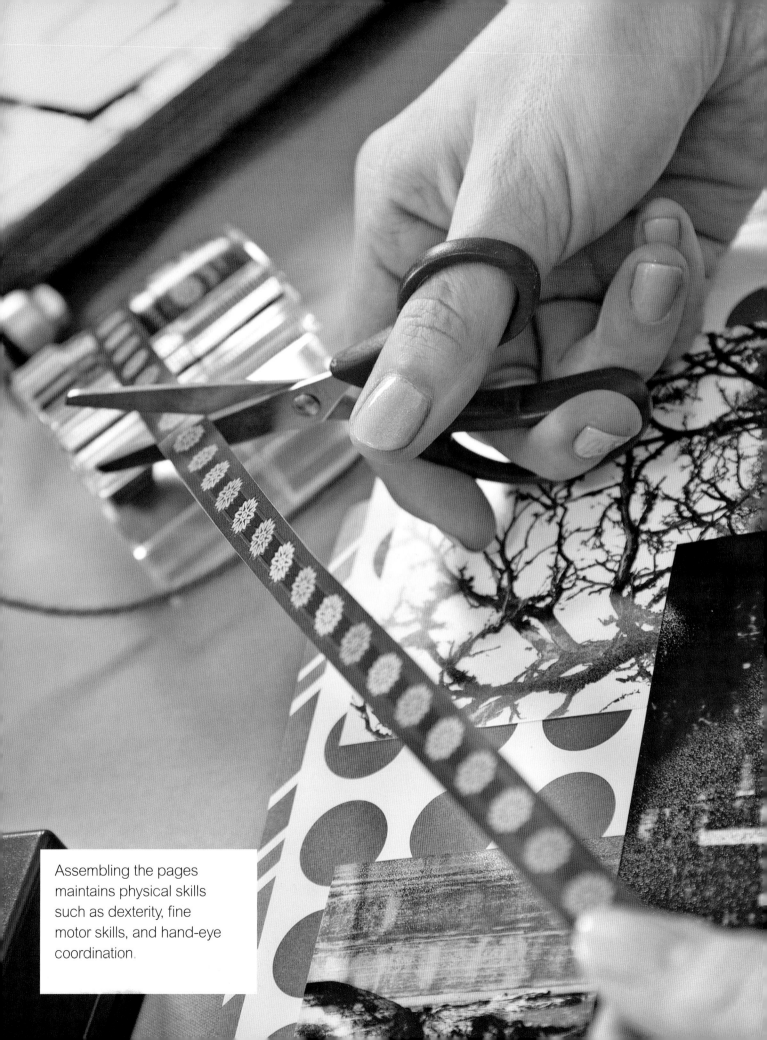

Assembling the pages maintains physical skills such as dexterity, fine motor skills, and hand-eye coordination.

The story of the telephone

The invention of the telephone by Alexander Graham Bell in the late 19th century began a revolution in society, opening up communication across the world. It was not until 1927 that calls were transmitted by radio waves, when the first call was made between New York and London. In the 1980s, technological advances made the first commercial cellular phones possible. The smartphone of today is actually a minicomputer.

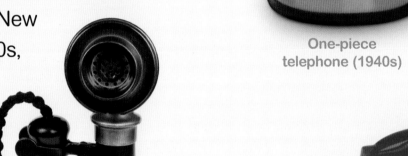

One-piece telephone (1940s)

Candlestick telephone (1900s)

Rotary-dial telephone (from 1930s)

TALK ABOUT…

What do you think Alexander Graham Bell would make of the impact his invention has had on the world?

Has the cell phone killed the art of conversation?

What can you do with your cell phone?

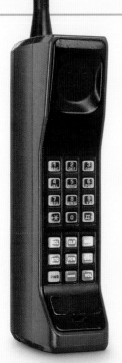

Cellular phone
(1980s)

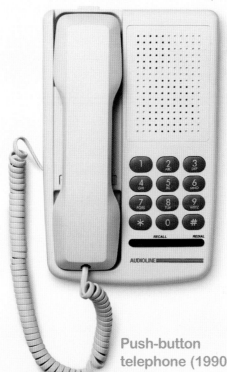

Push-button
telephone (1990s)

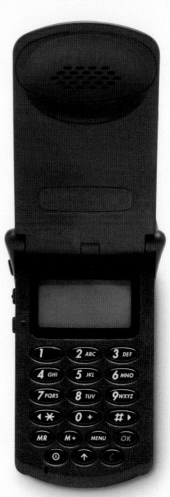

Flip phone (1990s)

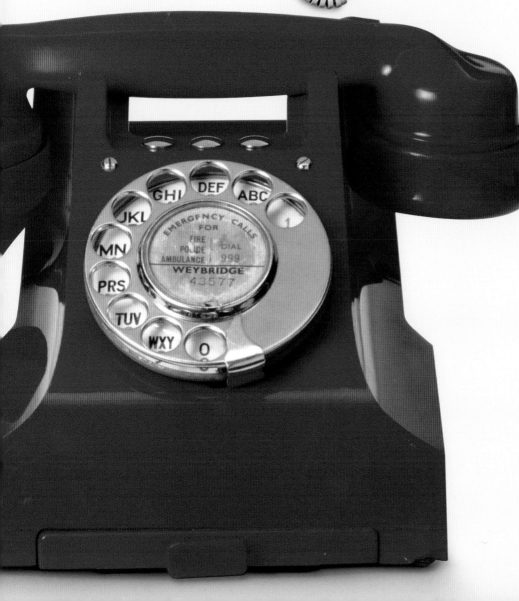

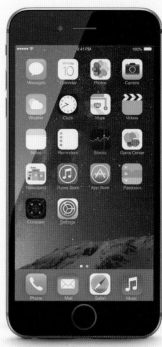

Smartphone (2010s)

Record your life story

Recording your life story can be very powerful, liberating, and affirming. It captures the unique history of your life to give others a true picture of who you are.

How to do it

You are the expert in your life story, so there is no right or wrong way to do it.

■ Gather memorabilia of your life. Sort it into chronological order and pick out the most significant items.

■ Talk to another person about the items you have collected, and write down the stories attached to them. It may be easier to talk generally rather than recall specific details.

■ You could use a template, with pages for life landmarks such as school days, relationships, working life, and hobbies.

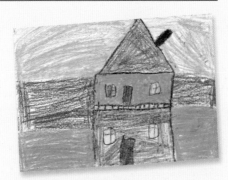

▲ You may want to include mementos such as your children's or grandchildren's artworks.

AT A GLANCE

✓ Sedentary

✓ 1 or 2 people

✓ Productivity

✓ 30–60 minutes at a time

✓ Moderately skilled

! May trigger negative as well as positive emotions

HOW IT HELPS

Recording your special life story can have a long-term, positive effect on mental well-being.

• Recalling significant life events (positive and negative) relies on long-term, episodic memory. Photographs, objects, or even smells help us to remember.

• Remembering challenging times is not always a bad thing—talking about them can be cathartic.

• Sharing our achievements in life increases confidence and self-esteem.

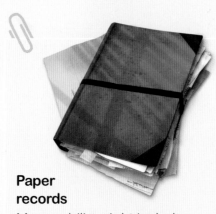

Paper records
Memorabilia might include paperwork, photographs, certificates, etc.

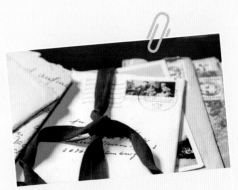

Mementos
Include anything flat enough to put in the book, such a lock of hair or old postcards.

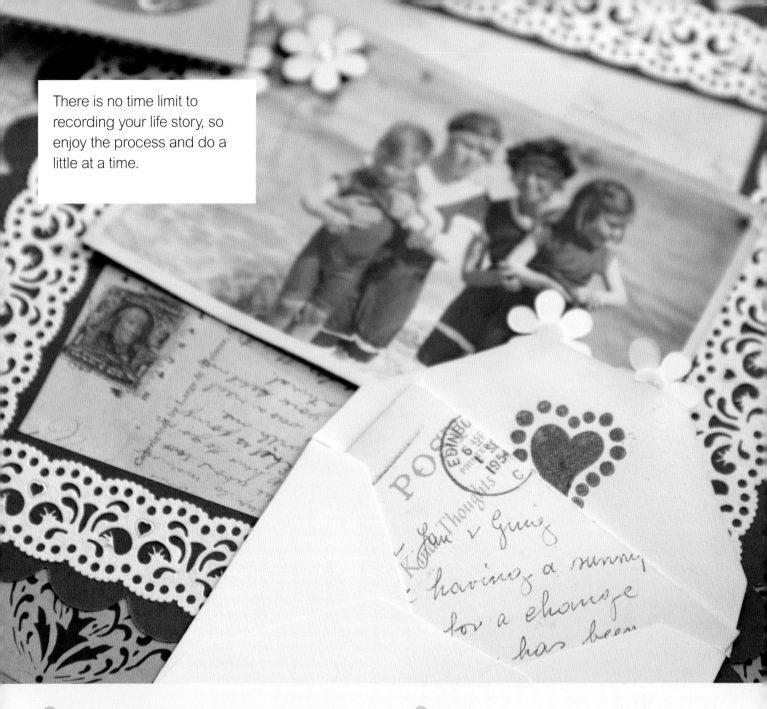

There is no time limit to recording your life story, so enjoy the process and do a little at a time.

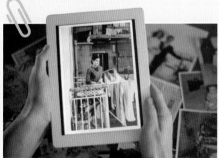

Digital resources
Go online to find a life-story template and images from the past, such as your old school.

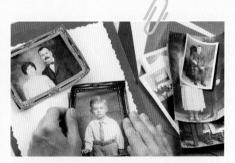

Create your book
Put the memorabilia in your life-story book, with the stories alongside each item.

Instead of a book, you could make a video or keep a memory box (see pages 88–89)

If you find the process emotionally difficult, try to express your feelings to another person

USEFUL TIPS

Make a theme bag

Fill a bag with items associated with pastimes or hobbies you have enjoyed. Handling these items will help you to recall your experiences, thoughts, and feelings from your past.

How to do it

Decide on a theme, based on your hobbies and interests, or on your experiences in the past.

■ Make a list of the things you could put in a bag. Check them off as you find them.

■ Choose a bag to suit the theme and place your chosen items in the bag. It is now ready to use.

■ Handle the items from your theme bag to recreate feelings and memories associated with them.

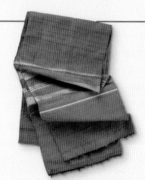

▲ If you cannot think of a theme, fill a rummage bag with things that are nice to touch, in a variety of shapes, sizes, colors, and textures.

HOW IT HELPS

Handling familiar objects stimulates the senses of sight, touch, and smell, which can trigger both emotional and episodic memories.

• Stimulating long-term memories in this way can encourage short-term memories.

• A theme bag can help to initiate a conversation, maintaining communication skills.

• Sharing experiences and achievements while talking about the objects increases self-esteem and a feeling of self-worth.

• There are no rules or any need for precision, so it is a fail-safe activity.

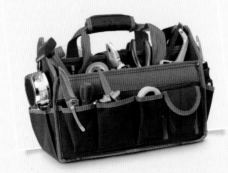

Toolbox
If you are a DIY enthusiast, you will enjoy handling your favorite tools and explaining how each tool is used.

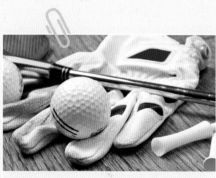

Sporting themes
If you were athletic in the past, fill a sports bag with pieces of gear, equipment, and trophies.

Handbag
Personal items such as gloves, lipstick, and jewelry in an old handbag could transport you back to events long ago.

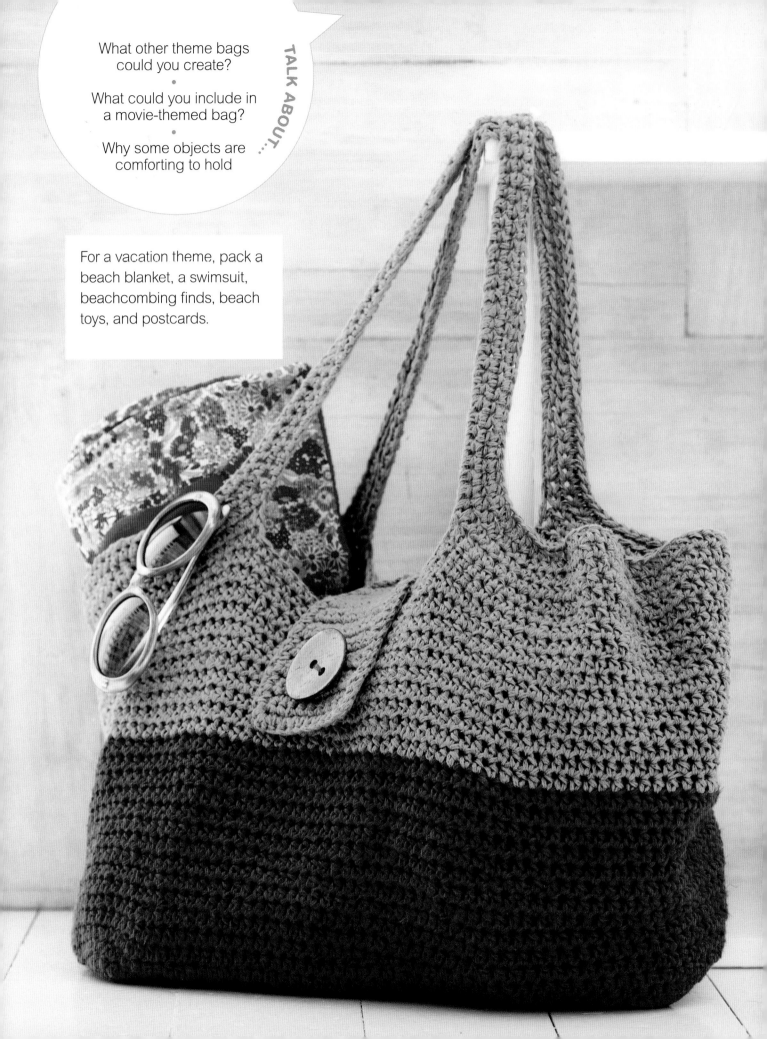

What other theme bags could you create?

What could you include in a movie-themed bag?

Why some objects are comforting to hold

TALK ABOUT...

For a vacation theme, pack a beach blanket, a swimsuit, beachcombing finds, beach toys, and postcards.

Watch an old movie

Whether spontaneous or planned, on your own or in the company of friends or family, watching a movie can transport you to another world.

How to do it

Rent or buy movies to watch on your TV or computer, take them out from the library, or go to a local theater.

■ Avoid violent or war movies, which might trigger negative emotional memories that you find difficult.

■ If concentrating is a challenge, avoid films with complex plots: musicals are a good choice.

■ If watching in company, take an break to discuss the movie so far: it will help with your concentration.

▶ There are many different genres to choose from. Old favorites are best at evoking memories of when you watched them and with whom.

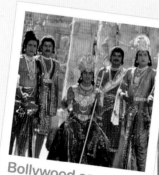
Bollywood sagas

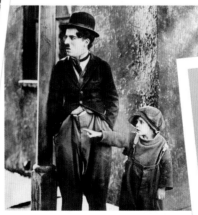
Silent era

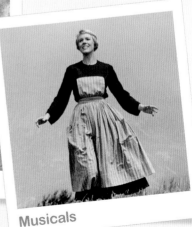
Musicals

Describe your favorite film
•
Did you ever copy a film star's hairstyle?
•
What makes a good cliffhanger?
•
Which films have produced famous quotations?

TALK ABOUT...

AT A GLANCE

✓ Sedentary

✓ 1 or more people

✓ Leisure

✓ 1½–2 hours

✓ Easy

HOW IT HELPS

Watching favorite films or home movies of family occasions and outings triggers emotional memories.

• Episodic memory may enable you to recall familiar phrases or scenes when rewatching a familiar film.

• Following a plot requires attention and concentration. Choose a time of day when you are alert, to benefit most.

• Enjoying and laughing along to a good comedy releases endorphins into the body and improves mood.

• Watching a movie with others creates a chance to socialize and share memories.

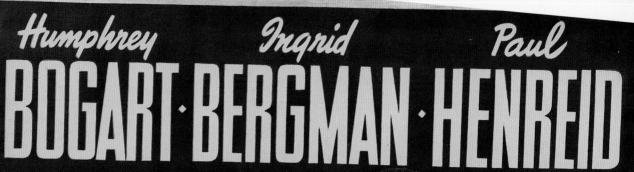

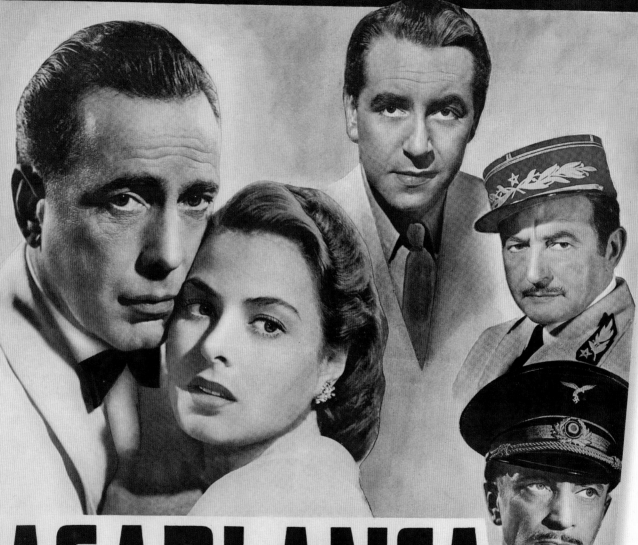

Some theaters now run showings of old movies without lengthy and distracting trailers.

Make caramel corn

Caramel corn is easy to make, but does involve the use of hot oil and boiling sugar, so take care. You may wish to ask for help with some steps. This recipe takes less than 10 minutes and makes enough for a large bowl.

WHAT YOU NEED

- Large saucepan with a lid
- Medium saucepan
- Wooden spoon
- Large mixing bowl
- Serving bowls or individual cartons

RECIPE INGREDIENTS

- 2 tbsp cooking oil
- ½ cup (100 g) popping corn
- 4 tbsp (50 g) butter
- ¼ cup (50 g) dark brown sugar, packed
- 3 tbsp (75 ml) corn syrup

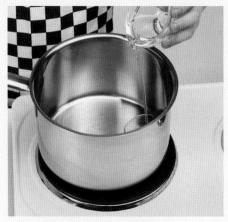

1 Pour the oil into the saucepan and add just 3 or 4 kernels of corn. Then place the lid on the pan.

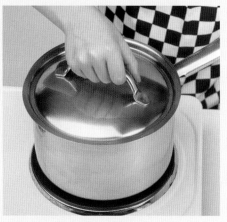

2 Heat over a low to moderate heat until all the kernels have popped. The oil is now hot enough.

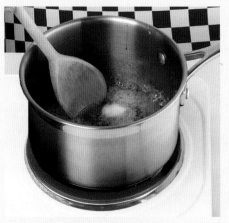

6 Put the butter, sugar, and syrup in another saucepan. Bring to a boil and cook for 2 minutes, stirring constantly.

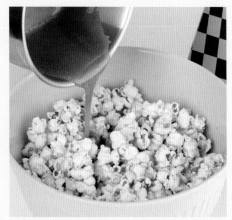

7 Turn off the heat. Transfer the popcorn into a large mixing bowl and pour the warm caramel sauce over it.

More popcorn flavors

Try making popcorn with different flavors. Follow steps 1 to 5, and instead of making caramel sauce, try adding grated cheese, dried herbs, melted chocolate, or maple syrup. Or, go for a classic taste, by sprinkling warm popcorn with salt or sugar, to taste, and stirring in 2 oz (50 g) of melted butter.

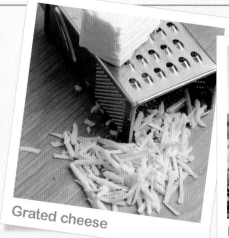

Grated cheese

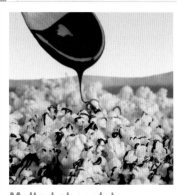

Melted chocolate

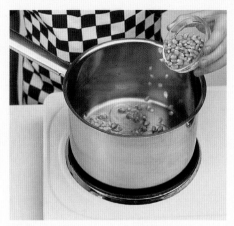

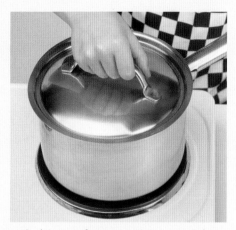

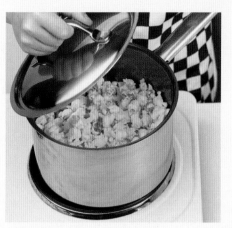

3 Remove the lid and quickly pour in all the corn kernels. Replace the lid and cook for a minute or so.

4 Listen for popping sounds as the kernels explode. Once they stop popping, gently shake the saucepan.

5 Turn off the heat. Remove the lid to let out the steam. Replace the lid and put the pan of popcorn to one side.

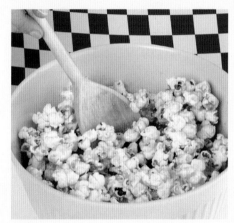

8 Stir the popcorn until the caramel sauce has cooled and is setting, so that it coats the popcorn evenly.

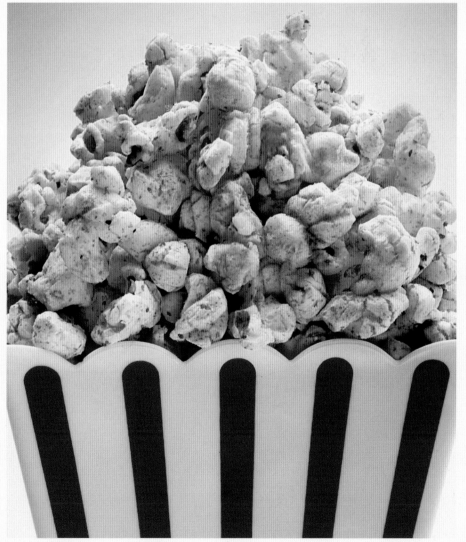

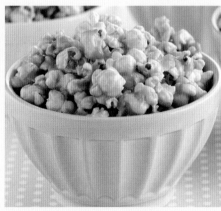

9 Leave the popcorn to cool. Then transfer to a serving bowl or cartons and enjoy.

▲ Using paper cartons for your popcorn makes watching an old movie more like a cinema outing.

MUSIC AND DANCE

Music provides a powerful means of connecting with other people, of exploring your memories, and of experiencing moments of joy. Bring more music into your life by playing an instrument if you can, or simply listen to your favorite music. Singing stimulates the entire brain, so even when words are becoming difficult, you can take pleasure in your innate ability to sing and respond to rhythm. Dancing also allows you to live in the moment and express yourself.

Do a dance

You might think of this as just a physical activity, but it may be a good exercise for the brain, and can enhance our memory.

How to do it

At the simplest level you can just put on some music and dance. If you want to learn a new dance or have fun with other people, join a class or get a friend who can dance to show you a few steps.

■ If you are not so good on your feet, consider chair-based activities.

■ If you're dancing at home, clear an area of the room and make sure there are no trip hazards.

▶ Dancing is a great social activity, whether you attend a formal event, an afternoon dance, or a class.

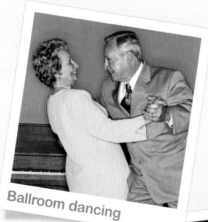
Ballroom dancing

Dancing partners
•
Your favorite dance styles
•
Musicals and films with dance sequences
•
Your recollections of dancing at special events

TALK ABOUT...

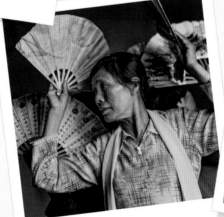
Folk dancing

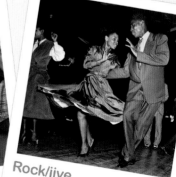
Rock/jive

HOW IT HELPS

Dancing involves coordination, thinking ahead (which helps creative thinking), and musicality. It also stimulates emotions.

• Learning dance steps helps to create new connections between brain cells, making the brain more resilient.

• If you have always danced, you use your procedural memory to dance familiar routines, reinforcing existing connections.

• The physical movements improve visual perception, balance, and spatial memory, and also release endorphins (feel-good hormones) into the brain.

• Dancing is a good way to express yourself, without the need to struggle for words.

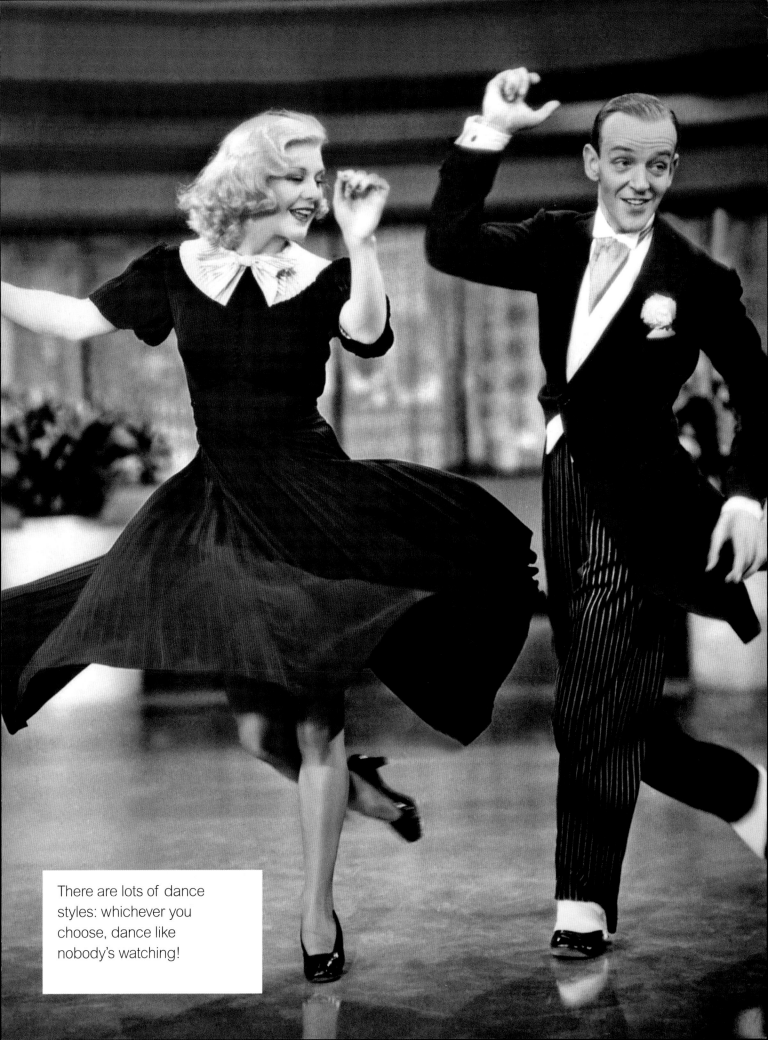

There are lots of dance styles: whichever you choose, dance like nobody's watching!

Listen to music

Listening to music is an easy way to stimulate the mind because it reaches parts of the brain that other forms of communication cannot.

How to do it

Music can be soothing or stimulating; your taste in listening may vary depending on the time of day.

■ Try listening to relaxing music before going to bed.

■ Singing, whistling, clapping, or tapping your feet are all ways of taking part—or you can just listen.

■ You may enjoy hymns and music from your place of worship.

■ You could listen to favorite songs and pieces of music by yourself, share them with others, or go to a concert.

AT A GLANCE

✓ Sedentary

✓ 1 or more people

✓ Leisure

✓ 30–60 minutes

✓ Easy

! May trigger powerful memories and feelings

HOW IT HELPS

Our ability to sing familiar songs and react to musical rhythms persists even after words become difficult.

• Music and songs from childhood and young adulthood often elicit vivid memories and help you to recall events, feelings, and people.

• Music enhances mood, and reduces anxiety and depression.

• Listening to music encourages us to move.

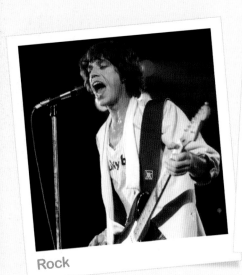

Rock

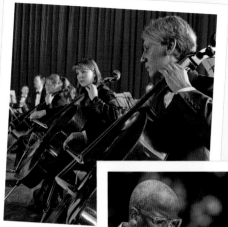

Classical

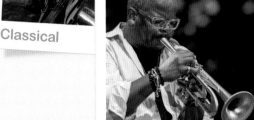

Jazz

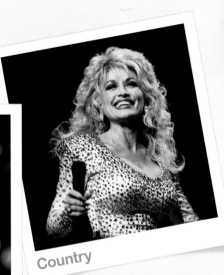

Country

▲ If you find that music you once enjoyed is too loud or has too fast a beat, try other types of music.

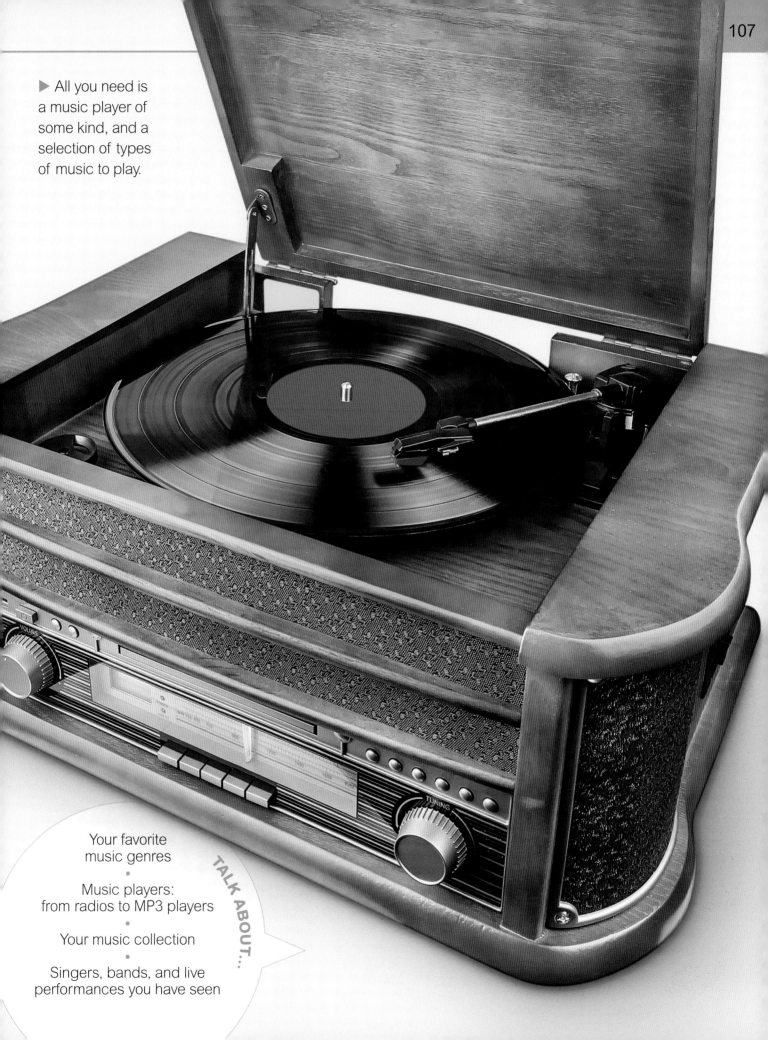

▶ All you need is
a music player of
some kind, and a
selection of types
of music to play.

Your favorite
music genres

Music players:
from radios to MP3 players

Your music collection

Singers, bands, and live
performances you have seen

TALK ABOUT...

Musicals

Musicals as a form of drama that incorporates dance and song into the story first became widely popular in the mid twentieth century. Hollywood film musicals like "Oklahoma!," "My Fair Lady", and "The Sound of Music" brought popular stage productions to a global audience. Theater and film musicals are still immensely popular around the world today.

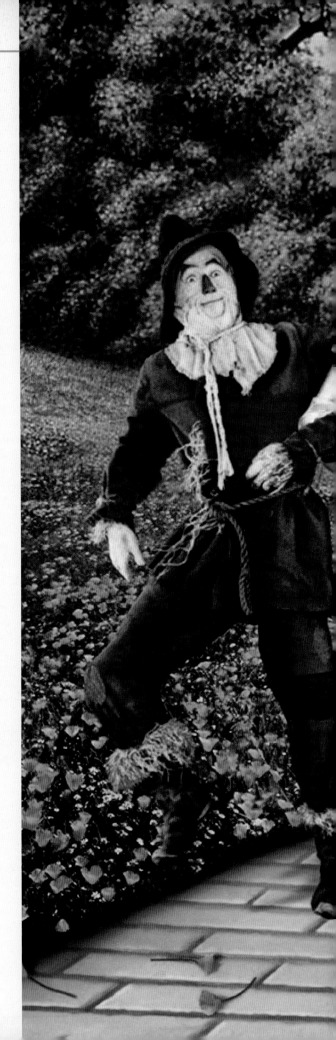

▶ The classic movie musical "The Wizard of Oz" was released in 1939. Here is Dorothy with the Scarecrow, Tin Man, and Cowardly Lion on the Yellow Brick Road.

Does music add to a story or interfere with it?

Which are best: modern musicals or old Hollywood blockbusters?

Which is your favorite musical?

TALK ABOUT...

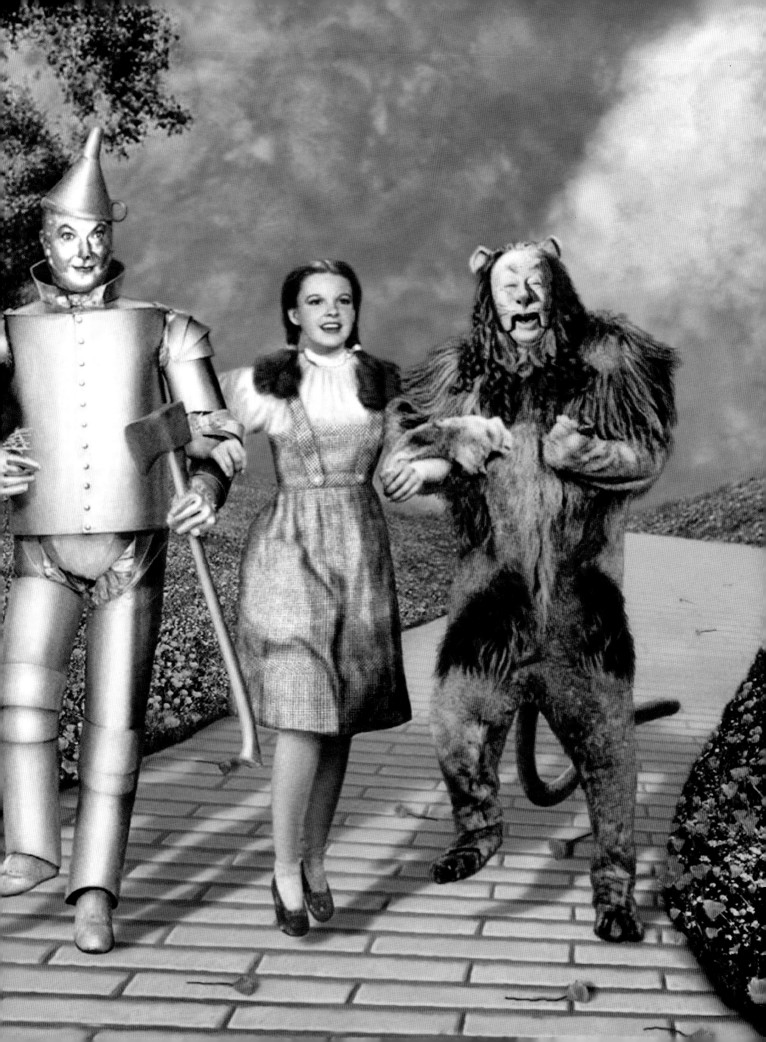

Create a playlist

Making it easier to find your favorite music will encourage you to listen more, so create your own lists of tracks or songs to suit different moods.

How to do it

Create one or more playlists of your favorite music. You can organize recordings by musical style or genre, alphabetically, or chronologically.

■ If you don't know how to create a digital playlist, get help from a family member or a how-to website.

■ Consider using online resources to download your favorite tunes.

■ Create the right ambience to listen to each playlist. Turn the lights low for relaxing music, or turn the sound up for uplifting music.

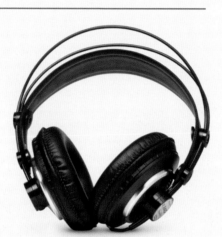

▲ Over-ear headphones help you to focus on the music and block out distracting background noises.

AT A GLANCE

✓ Sedentary

✓ 1 or more people

✓ Productivity/leisure

✓ Variable timeframe

✓ Variable difficulty

! May trigger negative emotions

HOW IT HELPS

Music can boost your mood, and help to maintain your sense of identity by reconnecting you with your earlier self and feelings from the time you first heard the music.

• Listening to familiar songs stimulates many different parts of the brain, including those responsible for memory, emotion, hearing, language, and rhythm.

• Organizing a playlist involves many cognitive skills—recognition, decision-making, initiation of tasks, and attentiveness.

Teenage idols

·

Live music events you attended

·

Acoustic music or rock and roll?

·

Your favorite singer or musician

TALK ABOUT...

▶ Dig out your music collection, whether on vinyl, CDs, cassette tapes, or on a phone, computer, or other digital device, to make your own playlists.

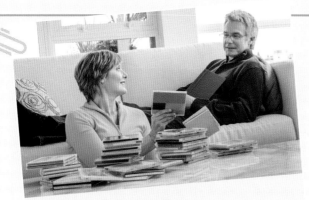

Choose your favorites
Listen to each album and make a note of your favorite tunes to add to a playlist.

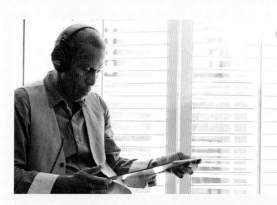

Mood music
Create playlists with different moods, such as one with relaxing music and one with energizing music.

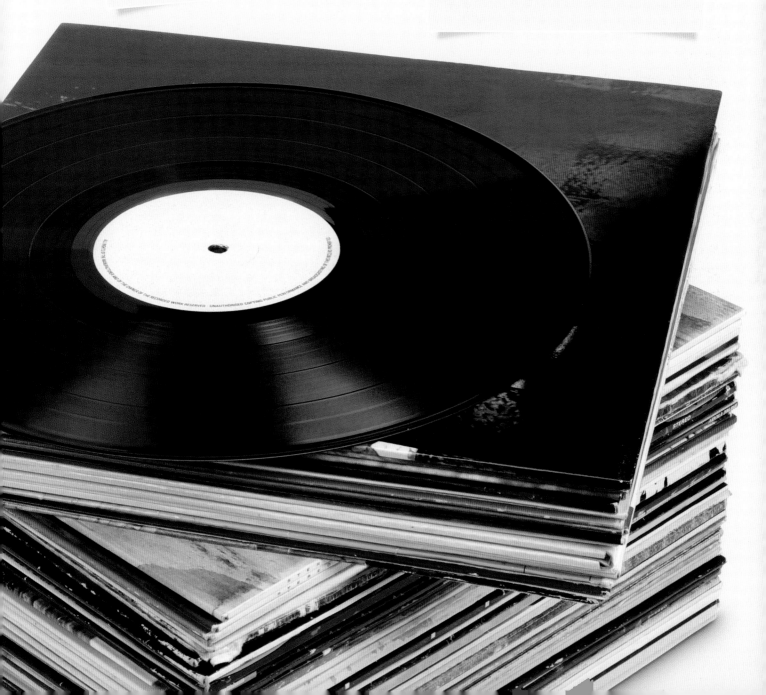

Singing is good for you

When words are becoming a struggle, the ability to sing remains. Even if your memory is unreliable, you will often remember the words and tunes of your favorite songs.

How to do it

There is no right or wrong way to sing. Do not worry whether you can hold a tune—just sing and enjoy yourself.

■ If you're unsure about joining a local choir, consider attending a singing group for people living with dementia. This will help you forge social bonds and keep you connected to others.

■ A karaoke screen provides the words, and can be used if you can't recall the lyrics.

AT A GLANCE

✓ Gentle activity

✓ 1 or more people

✓ Leisure

✓ Variable timeframe

✓ Easy

! May trigger powerful memories and feelings

HOW IT HELPS

The ability to sing and follow a rhythm is located in a different part of the brain than the part dealing with communication. Singing can strengthen connections between such areas and may improve communication.

• This activity is failure-free, so it can have a positive effect on your mood.

• Songs can evoke a powerful emotional memory of a moment in the past, aiding recall of details such as people, dates, and places.

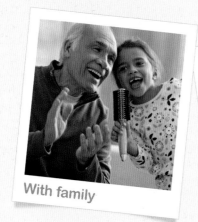

With family

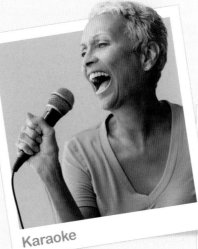

Karaoke

▼ Whether you do it in the shower, with family, or in a group, singing can lighten your mood.

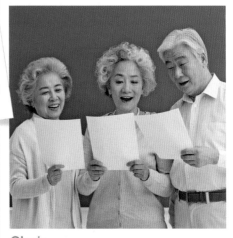

Choir

Songs from your place of worship

•

Songs that can be sung in rounds

•

Songs from around the world

TALK ABOUT...

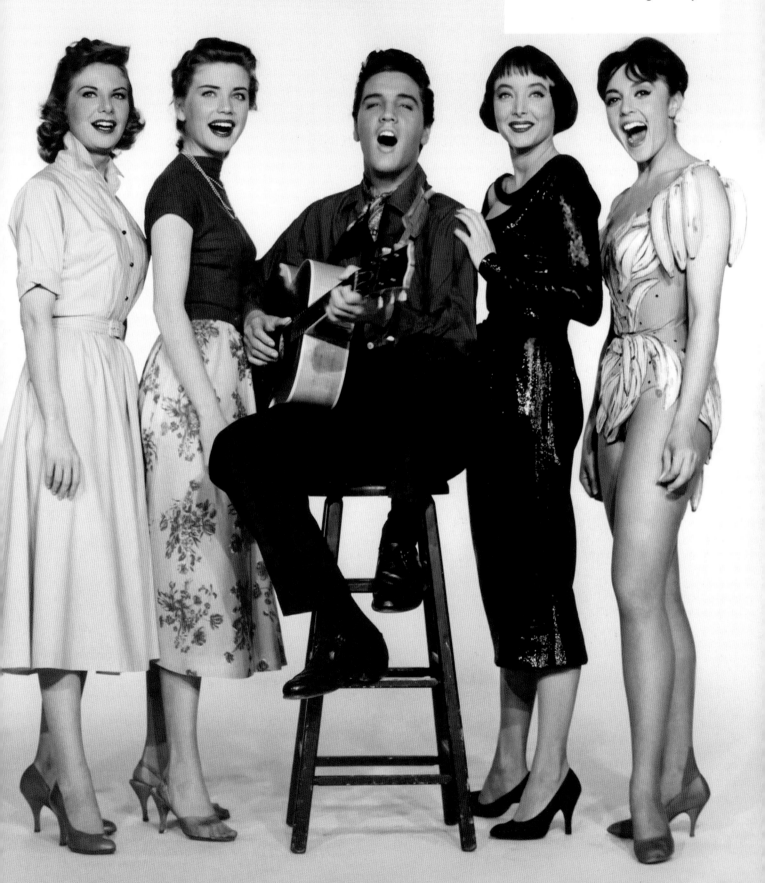

Sing along to familiar tunes or to recordings of your favorite singers to evoke memories of times gone by.

Play the musical journey game

In this game, you can enjoy a sing-along while you share memories of songs associated with significant milestones and activities in your life.

How to do it

Prepare some game cards: take about ten cards or pieces of paper and write one key life milestone, memorable event, or activity on them, such as a wedding.

■ Play the game with two to four players. The more players who join in, the more varied the song choices will be.

■ Give your imagination free rein, go with the theme, and you may be surprised at how many songs you can recall.

■ This is not a memory test. If you forget some of the words, hum along.

AT A GLANCE
✓ Sedentary
✓ 2 or more people
✓ Leisure
✓ Variable timeframe
✓ Easy

HOW IT HELPS
The musical journey game provides prompts for players to recall memories, such as childhood, a favorite vacation, and family festivities.

• The game should be spontaneous and fun, and is good for your sense of well-being.

• Comparing your choices with family and friends is a good conversation starter and helps you to be socially active, which encourages brain vitality.

• There are no wrong answers or time limits, so you can enjoy practicing your recall without any pressure to get it right.

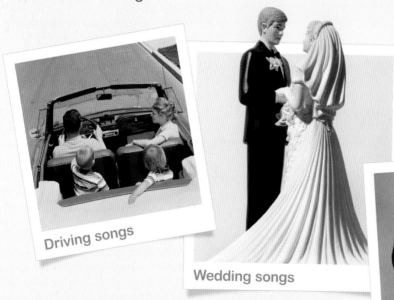

Driving songs

Wedding songs

Lullabies

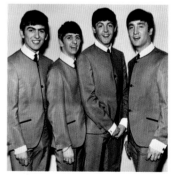

Pop idols

▲ Here are some more ideas for categories for your game cards.

The rules of the musical journey game

TALK ABOUT...

Do you have songs that are linked to special moments or events in your life?

•

Describe the qualities of a classic song

•

What songs always make you feel happy?

■ Pick a card and think of a song to match. Sing the first line or chorus of the song.

■ Take turns thinking of a song to match the same category, and sing a bit of the song you remember.

■ Other players can join in the song if they want.

■ When you can think of no more songs in that category, choose another card.

■ Play the game for as long as you want. You may find that you do not even get past the first card.

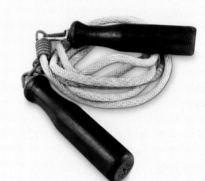

Songs from school

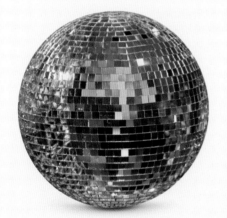

Songs to dance to

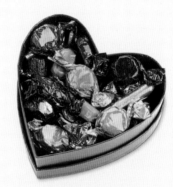

Love songs

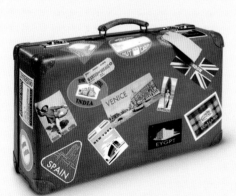

Vacation songs

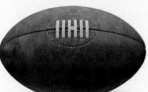

Sports songs

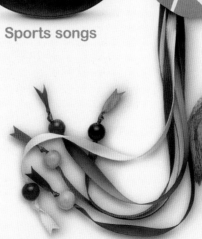

Songs for festivals

▶ If you don't want to make cards, use these examples of song categories for your game.

Play an instrument

Playing an instrument benefits your brain more than simply listening to music, and it does not matter if you're an accomplished musician or an avid novice.

How to do it

Whether you play alone or in a group, the key is to enjoy creating music, so adapt the level of participation to your ability.

■ It is never too late to learn how to play an instrument. Choose a relatively easy one, such as the ukulele.

■ If playing is too challenging, try tapping on a drum or table top or clapping along to familiar tunes.

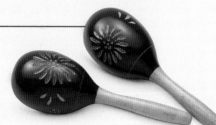

▲ Percussion instruments such as maracas, bells, cymbals, and castanets are great ways to make music.

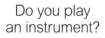

Guitar

AT A GLANCE

✓ Gentle activity

✓ 1 or more people

✓ Leisure

✓ Variable timeframe

✓ Variable difficulty

HOW IT HELPS

The area of the brain that interprets music and recognizes rhythm may remain intact longer than some other brain parts.

• Evidence suggests that playing an instrument can delay cognitive decline.

• Playing an instrument makes different parts of your brain work together, maintaining those connections.

• Attention levels increase, which improves cognition and memory recall.

• Practicing regularly helps to retain your musical skill and keeps you physically active by using fine or gross motor skills (depending upon your instrument).

◀ Whatever instrument you play, participating in music-making benefits you more than simply listening.

Do you play an instrument?

•

Describe some different groups of instruments

•

Orchestra or big band— which is your favorite?

TALK ABOUT...

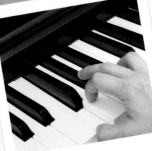

Piano

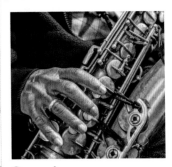

Saxophone

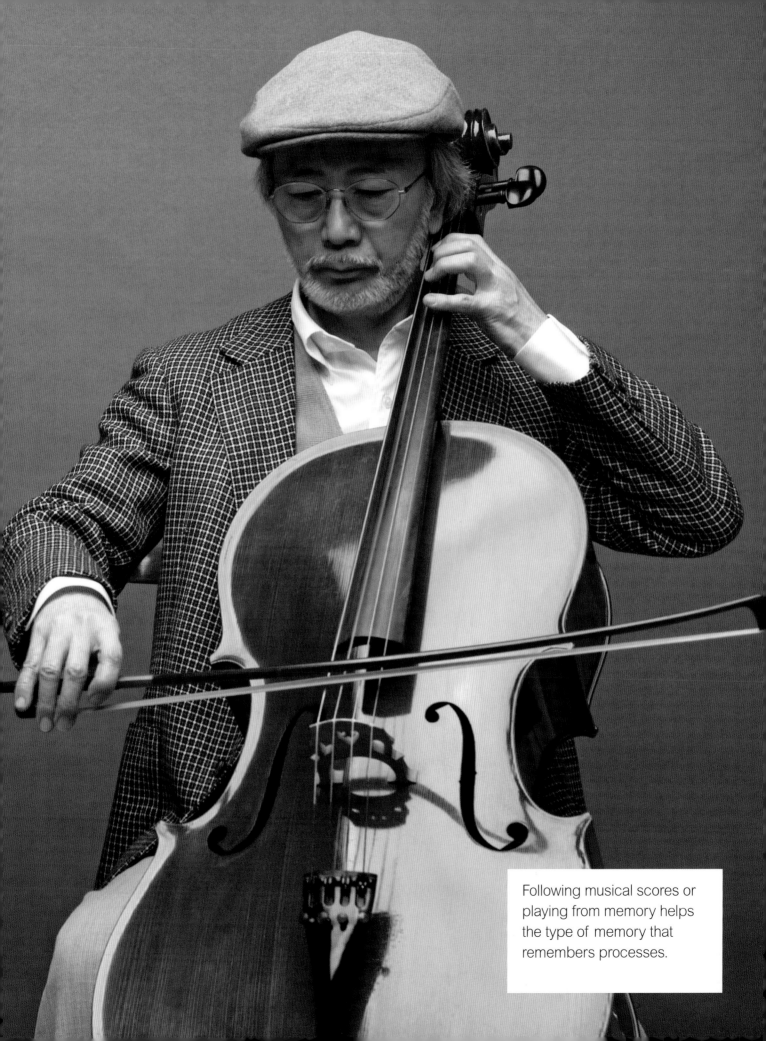

Following musical scores or playing from memory helps the type of memory that remembers processes.

PUZZLES AND GAMES

Stimulating the mind with puzzles and games is thought to boost your ability to think, reason, concentrate, and deal with tasks. There is some truth in the "use it or lose it" argument, and exercising your brain may increase brain health. Choosing a suitable game or puzzle is key. It should be challenging enough to keep you interested and make you think, but not so hard that you get frustrated.

Do a jigsaw puzzle

This very popular pastime provides an enjoyable challenge; the more pieces of the puzzle there are, the more demanding it will be. You could do it alone or work in a team, with each person taking on a section.

How to do it

You'll need a flat area to work on, at which you can sit comfortably for a while.

■ Empty the contents of the box on to the work area. If there are lots of pieces, you may want to take out only some of them at a time; too many on the table might be confusing.

■ Turn all pieces picture-side up. Sort them into similar groups before you start.

■ Work on small sections at a time.

■ Put all the edge pieces in one pile. If some of the remaining pieces clearly belong together, sort those pieces into their own pile.

■ Make sure all the pieces are easy for you to see and find on the table.

■ Assemble the edge pieces first—that makes a frame to work within.

▲ Sorting pieces into piles of similar colors makes it easier to do the puzzle.

AT A GLANCE

✓ Sedentary

✓ 1 or 2 people

✓ Leisure

✓ Variable timeframe

✓ Easy

HOW IT HELPS

Solving jigsaw puzzles works and connects both sides of the brain, as well as connections between brain cells. This can help to maintain your ability to understand, to learn, and to remember.

• The visual element enhances visual perception and spatial processing in the brain.

• Handling and placing the pieces correctly exercises the parts of the brain involved with motor skills and coordination.

• Matching the pieces stimulates the brain to retain information about shapes and colors. Repeating this activity helps short-term memory.

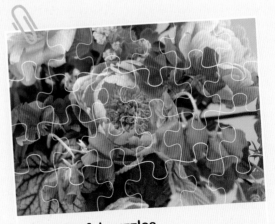

Meaningful puzzles
Completing a puzzle that ties in with an interest, like gardening, can be even more rewarding.

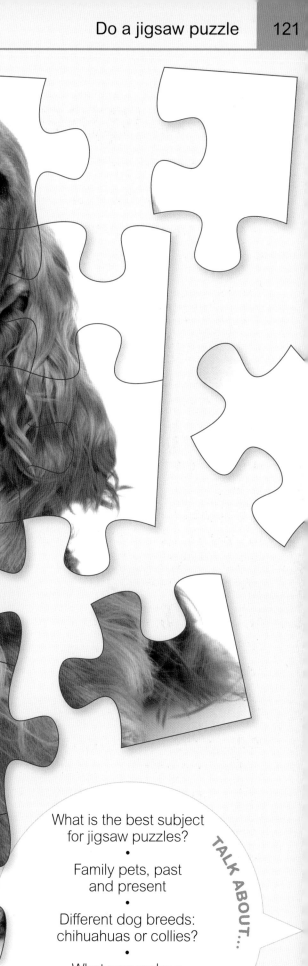

TALK ABOUT...

What is the best subject for jigsaw puzzles?

•

Family pets, past and present

•

Different dog breeds: chihuahuas or collies?

•

What can make a puzzle difficult?

Make a jigsaw puzzle

Making your own jigsaw puzzle means that you have more pictures to choose from and you can make it as easy or as difficult as you like.

Choose a picture

You can choose any subject that interests you, but a picture that has some personal meaning may hold your interest longer.

■ Consider the difficulty level of the picture itself. Lots of areas with little or no detail will make the puzzle more difficult to do.

■ Pictures with well-defined shapes and good contrasts of color will make the puzzle easier to do.

■ Look for pictures of familiar things: they are easier to imagine and reassemble after the puzzle is broken apart and jumbled up.

■ There are companies that can turn your favorite photographs into jigsaws puzzles. Get help to search for them online if you need to.

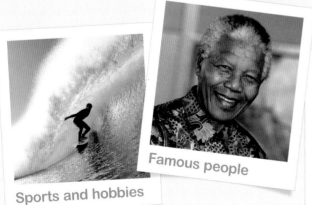
Sports and hobbies

Famous people

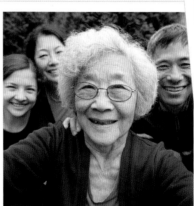
Friends and family

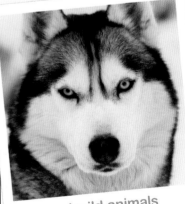
Pets and wild animals

▲ You can find pictures in magazines, photos, postcards, old calendars, and online.

AT A GLANCE

✓ Sedentary

✓ 1 or 2 people

✓ Productivity/leisure

✓ 30–60 minutes

✓ Easy

! Involves use of scissors

HOW IT HELPS

From choosing a picture to cutting things out, there are a number of skills involved in this activity.

• Choosing a picture engages the brain and stimulates the emotions. Memories can play a part here, with recall of past events, places, and people.

• Planning an activity and remembering the steps uses short-term memory.

• Dexterity and coordination are involved in drawing and cutting.

Choose a cutting pattern

More pieces make the puzzle more difficult, so choose a pattern that gives you just enough of a challenge, and is not too hard or easy. Also think about what shapes you can easily cut.

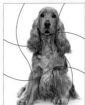
Large squares

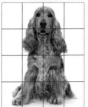
Wavy lines

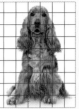
Small squares

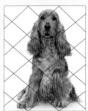
Diamonds

How to do it

Once you have your picture, get all your equipment together and follow these easy steps. Remember to let the glue set before you start cutting up the picture. Simpler puzzles with fewer pieces can be quick and fun to make and to do.

WHAT YOU NEED
- Ruler
- Thick, black marker
- Your picture
- Scissors
- Glue stick
- Piece of cardboard

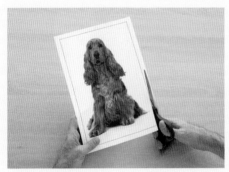

1 Use a ruler and pen to draw straight sides around the picture. Cut out the picture along the lines you have drawn.

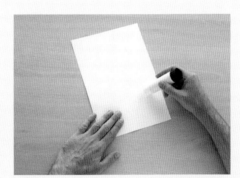

2 Turn the picture over and spread an even layer of glue on the back. Take care to cover it completely.

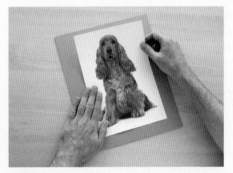

3 Lay the picture on a piece of sturdy cardboard that is larger than the picture. Press the picture firmly on the cardboard.

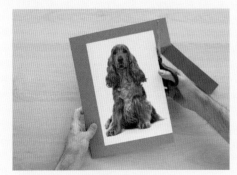

4 Use a pair of scissors to trim off the excess cardboard, cutting carefully around the picture.

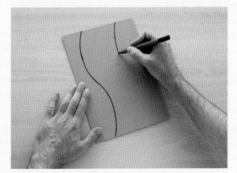

5 Turn the cardboard over and use a thick, black marker to draw your chosen cutting pattern on the back.

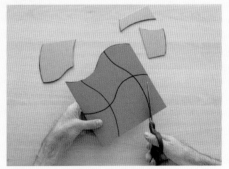

6 Once the glue has completely dried, cut out the pieces following the lines you drew on the back.

Test your nose and taste buds

Both smell and taste are very powerful senses and stimulating them regularly is great exercise for your brain.

How to do it

Make the most of every opportunity to stimulate your senses of smell and taste.

■ In the kitchen, experiment with new flavors. Try comparing the taste of a familiar fruit or herb with a more exotic or less familiar one.

■ Taste herbs, fruits, and vegetables you have grown.

■ In your home, enjoy smells such as fresh laundry, furniture polish, or shampoo.

HOW IT HELPS

Smell and taste are strongly linked to emotional memory. Sensory input from the nose—involved in both smell and taste—travels directly to the brain's emotional center, which has an important role in memory recall.

• Talking about those memories helps you to feel connected and uses your communication skills.

• Stimulating the senses can reduce agitation and restlessness, and improve sleep.

• Tasting food or drinks from your younger days can evoke strong memories.

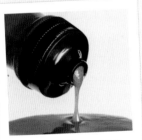
Spicy chili sauce

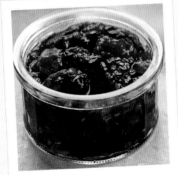
Sweet jam

TALK ABOUT...

Describe your favorite smells and tastes

•

Which animal has the best sense of smell?

•

Do you love or hate the smell of tar?

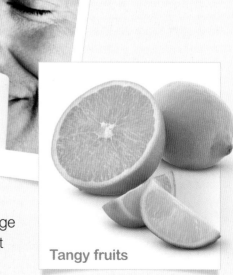
Fragrant coffee

Tangy fruits

▲ Relish the taste of your food; you could also challenge your taste buds by trying out new flavor experiences.

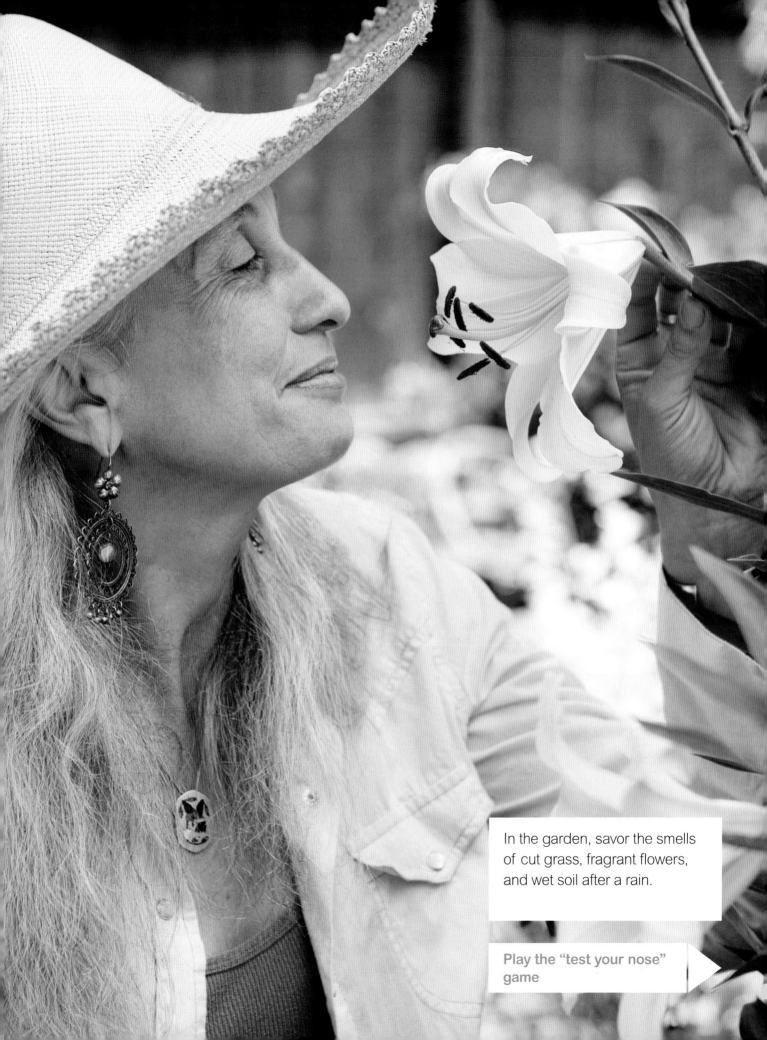

In the garden, savor the smells of cut grass, fragrant flowers, and wet soil after a rain.

Play the "test your nose" game ➤

Play the "Test Your Nose" game

Put your senses to the test by playing a smelling game: you try to identify and recognize the smell of different substances without seeing them. It is stimulating as well as a lot of fun.

How to do it

Prepare 6–12 strongly smelling items, each one in a container. Make answer cards that each show a picture of one item.

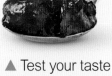

▲ Test your taste buds too, by getting a friend to put different edible substances on teaspoons and tasting each one with your eyes closed.

■ To play the game, place the answer cards in a row on a table. Close your eyes or wear a blindfold to smell each container in turn. Place each container on the answer card that corresponds to its smell.

■ You may prefer not to use cards, but just to try to recognize various smells.

HOW IT HELPS

Smell memories can evoke different emotions. For example, the smell of baby powder may bring back memories of a child.

• You will use a range of cognitive skills in preparing and playing the game, including concentration, recognition, and decision-making. It can help with word retrieval too.

• This game is an opportunity for fun and laughter. Socially engaging in this way can lift your mood and well-being.

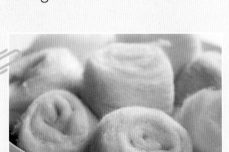

Smelly liquids
To make a smelling sample from a liquid, such as vinegar or wine, soak a cotton ball with a small amount.

Smelling containers
Place each sample in a small, opaque container with a lid. Players should not see the samples.

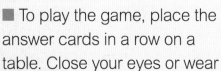

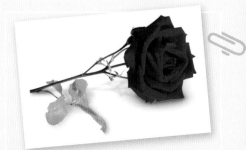

Make answer cards
Glue a cut-out or printed image onto an index card to make each answer card.

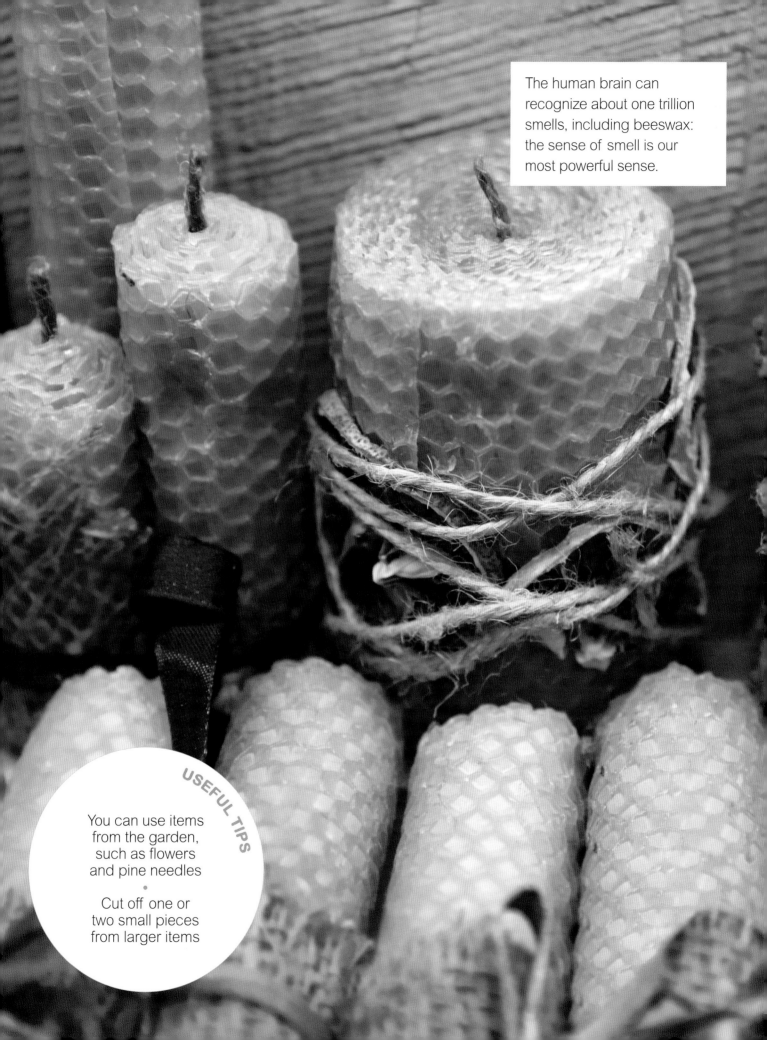

The human brain can recognize about one trillion smells, including beeswax: the sense of smell is our most powerful sense.

USEFUL TIPS

You can use items from the garden, such as flowers and pine needles

·

Cut off one or two small pieces from larger items

Play a word game

There is a huge variety of word games to enjoy, either on your own, such as crosswords, or with others, such as hangman.

How to do it

Be spontaneous. Not all word games need to be structured or planned; do them when you feel like it, not as an exercise.

■ You could simplify your favorite puzzles by choosing less complex equivalents. For example, rather than trying to solve a word-search grid of 20 x 20 letters, look for one with 10 x 10 letters.

■ Use magnetic letters to solve an anagram or rearrange a random selection of seven letters to create as many words as you can.

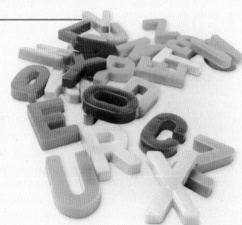

▲ Magnetic letters can be fun: put them on the fridge and do a word puzzle, a little bit at a time.

HOW IT HELPS

A highly complex and organized archiving system is used to store different word groups in various areas of the brain, so your entire brain is active when searching for a word.

• Engaging in stimulating activities like word games can benefit the brain. Word games help to practice word retrieval, which can also help maintain communication skills and slow down cognitive decline.

USEFUL TIPS

Choose a game at a level that suits your changing needs

•

Do not think of word games as a test—the stress will make it harder to retrieve words

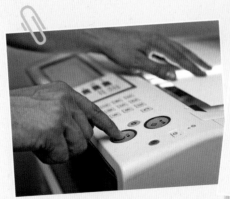

Photocopy puzzles
Make word puzzles easier to see by enlarging them on a copier machine.

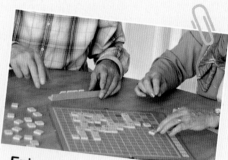

Enjoy a shared game
Have fun playing word games with family and friends or solving a word puzzle together.

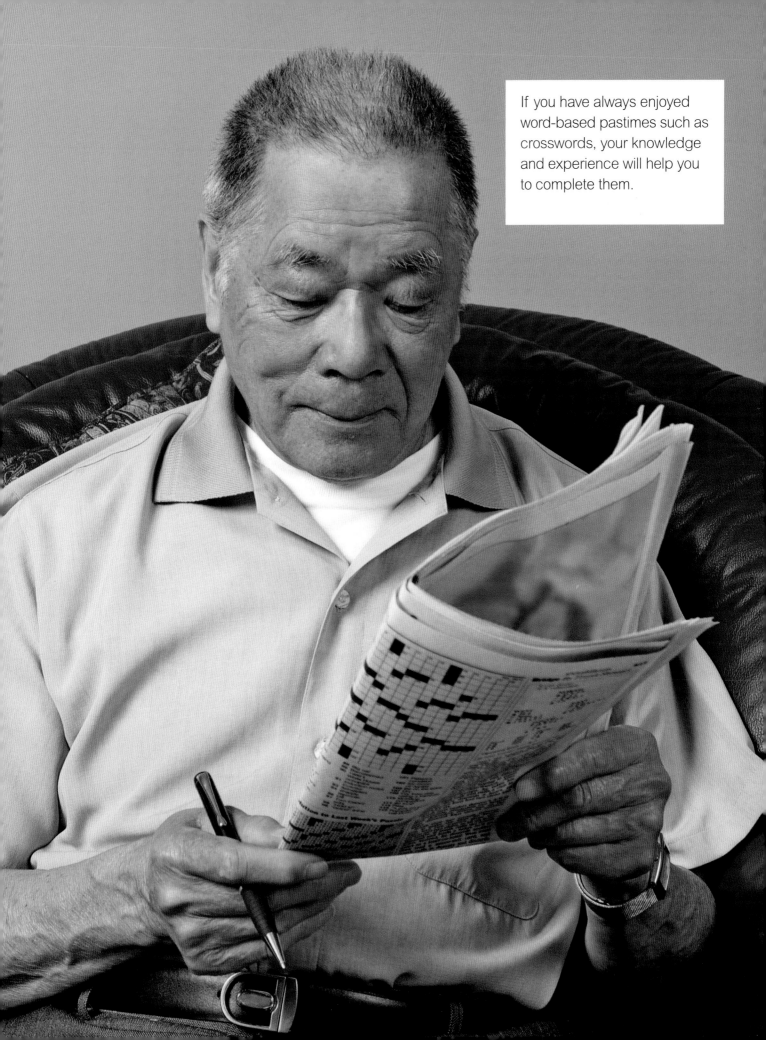

If you have always enjoyed word-based pastimes such as crosswords, your knowledge and experience will help you to complete them.

Play the word chain game

This game is a stress-free, fun way of using your memory and rehearsing your word retrieval.

How to do it

The more people who join you to play the word chain game, the more random and fun it will be.

■ You may find it easier to have no more than four players to limit the amount of information to process.

■ This is not a memory test. You do not need to recall all the words in the chain, only the last word spoken.

■ You can play the game for as long as you want. Simply stop when you have had enough.

HOW IT HELPS

There are no wrong answers in this game, so you can enjoy practicing your word recall without any pressure to get it right. This slows decline and helps you to feel positive about yourself.

• When we learn words, we organize and store them by category in specific parts of the brain, but use the entire brain to find them. If you think of Australia, you may unlock other words in the category of place names.

• Playing the game involves being socially active, which can help to maintain brain vitality and reduce stress.

• There is no time pressure with this game—players can find words at their own pace.

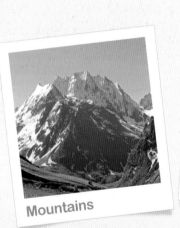
Mountains

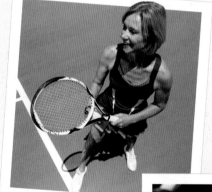
Tennis

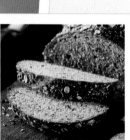
Bread

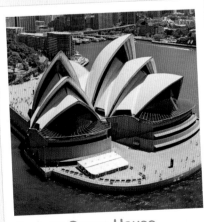
Sydney Opera House

▲ Here are some more ideas for words to start your word chain game.

The rules of the game

■ To start, one person says a word.

■ The next person says a word that is associated in some way to the first word.

■ The third person thinks of a third, connected word, and so on.

■ The word chain can be as long as you like. If the chain is broken, simply choose a new word and start again.

Complete the names of famous couples—for example Fred Astaire and ?

•

Think of opposite words— for example "up" and "down"

•

Do you know any tongue twisters?

TALK ABOUT...

▶ Here is an example of a word chain beginning with "bird."

Can you think of the next word?

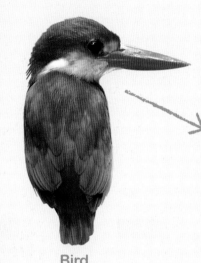
Bird

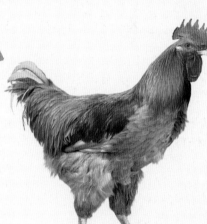
Chicken

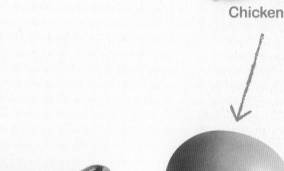
Egg

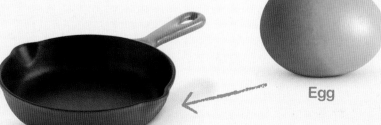
Frying pan

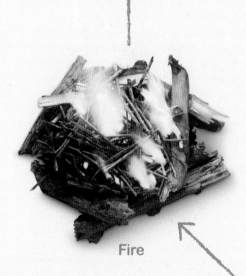
Fire

Moon landings

On July 20, 1969, millions watched around the world as the spacecraft Apollo 11 landed on the moon. The next day, Neil Armstrong and Buzz Aldrin were the first humans to step on the surface of the moon. Armstrong's famous first words began with the phrase, "One small step for [a] man…" In the years since, space travel has become a regular event, and modern society now depends heavily upon space technology such as communications satellites.

▶ This Apollo 16 mission to the moon took place in April 1972. Two astronauts landed in the small module "Orion," seen here behind their lunar vehicle.

Could space tourism happen?

If you could travel to the moon, would you go?

Or would you rather gaze at the stars from the safety of the Earth?

TALK ABOUT...

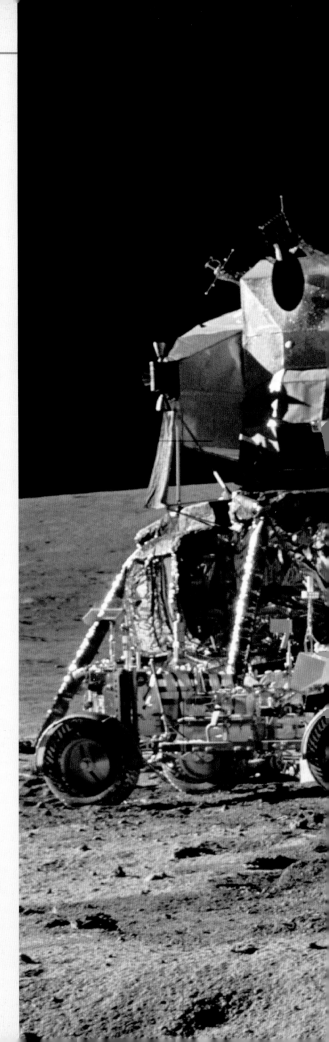

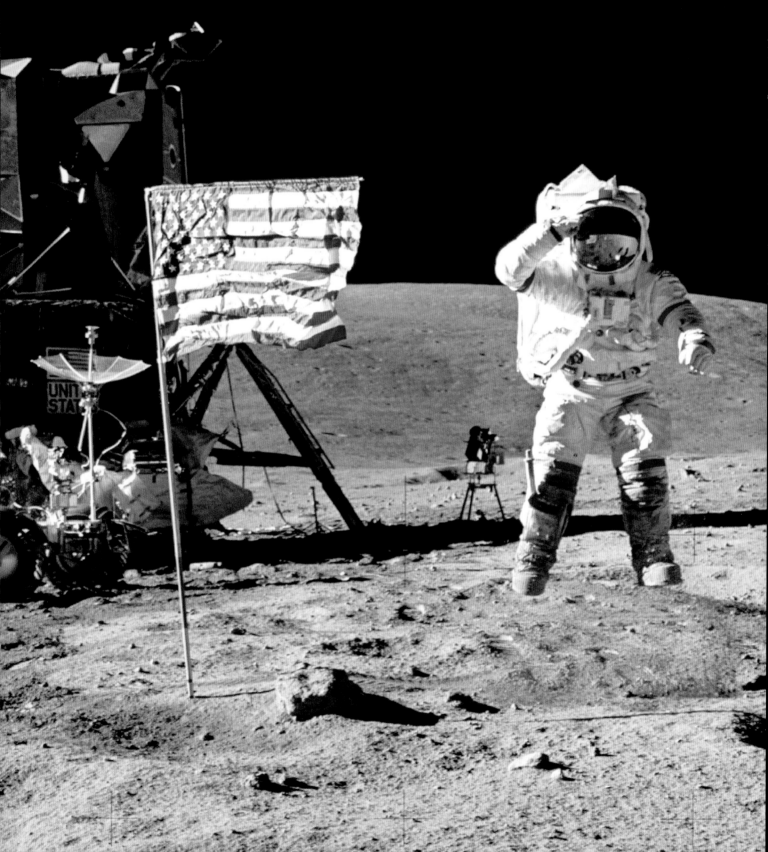

Play with numbers

You may find number games appeal to you more than word games, whether you do them on your own or with friends.

How to do it

Complete a game in your own time, and in stages, if you want. Don't put pressure on yourself to complete it in the quickest time.

■ Simplify a game by reducing the number of options, such as fewer possible answers or smaller grids.

■ Darts is a wonderful way to use maths skills. You could practice alone or in a team. Try playing "Around the clock": you have to get number 1, then 2, and so on, until you reach number 20.

▶ There are a lot of ways in which you can enjoy using numbers, from solving puzzles to playing sports in which you need to keep score.

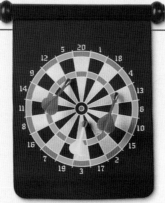

▲ A dartboard that uses magnetic darts rather than standard sharp ones is safer.

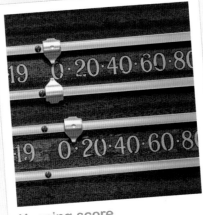

Keeping score

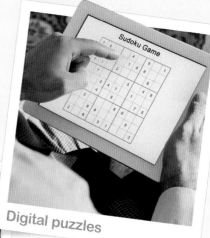

Digital puzzles

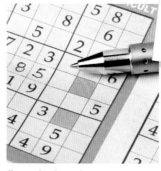

Puzzle book

TALK ABOUT...

Other number games you enjoy

•

Which do you prefer: numbers or words?

•

Jobs that require good maths skills

HOW IT HELPS

Games and puzzles that involve numbers help to keep your brain active, specifically areas of the temporal lobe, close to the ear, that are also involved in language skills.

• Playing with numbers may help to maintain cognitive skills such as logical thinking, reasoning, problem-solving, concentration, and attention.

• Completing games with family and friends adds a social element, which can reduce stress and anxiety, lower blood pressure, alleviate loneliness and depression, and improve sleep.

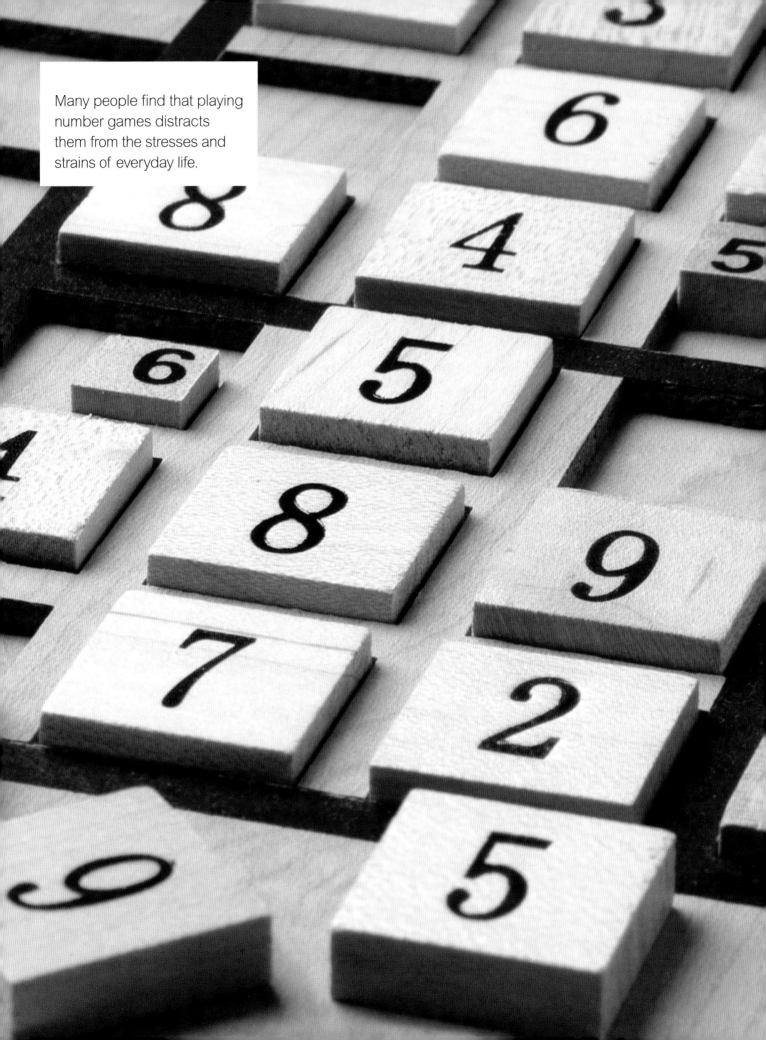

Many people find that playing number games distracts them from the stresses and strains of everyday life.

Play bingo

Bingo is an enjoyable game that also keeps the brain active. It can be easily adapted to suit players of any level.

How to do it

Whether you are playing bingo in a social club or with family or friends, follow these basic steps.

■ Nominate one person as the bingo caller and give each player a bingo card and counters.

■ The caller calls out one number at a time. Ask the bingo caller to hold up a laminated sheet of paper, with each number on it, at the same time to make it easier.

■ If any player has that number on their card, they place a chip on it. Once a player has a complete row of chips, they call out "Bingo!" and the caller checks the card.

■ You could make or buy bingo cards or download and print them from online websites.

HOW IT HELPS

Being sociable and laughing together releases endorphins (feel-good hormones), boosting the immune system, relieving stress, and reducing pain.

• Focusing on the numbers being called and recognizing and marking them on a card involves many cognitive skills, including interpreting and understanding speech, and translating comprehension into action.

• Playing bingo can help to maintain hand-eye coordination and dexterity.

• Bingo combines social and mental stimulation, which reduces anxiety and depression.

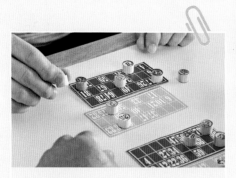

Smaller-grid bingo cards
Bingo cards with fewer squares make the game less complex.

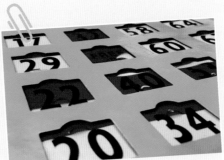

Shutter bingo cards
Shutter cards can also be used. Just change the paper cards inside for a new game.

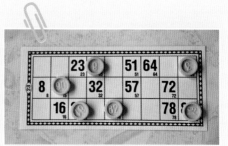

Fewer numbers
Some bingo cards have blank squares and fewer numbers, which makes it easier to play.

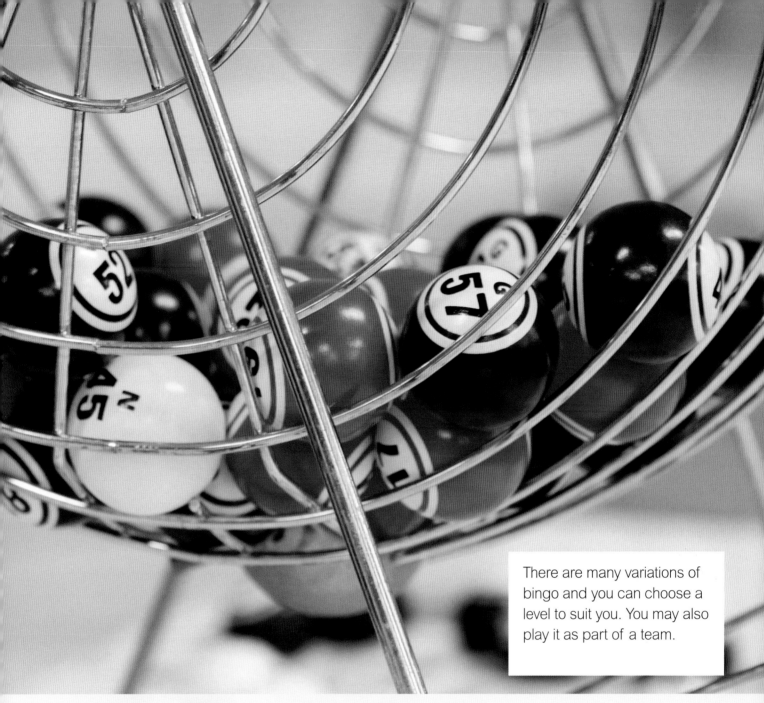

There are many variations of bingo and you can choose a level to suit you. You may also play it as part of a team.

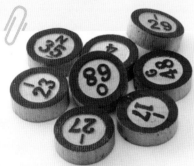

Large counters
If bingo counters are getting difficult to handle, try using larger cork-style counters.

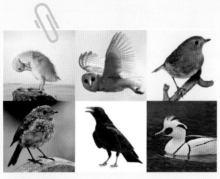

Picture bingo
Bingo cards may have themed pictures. Match each card to one the bingo caller holds up.

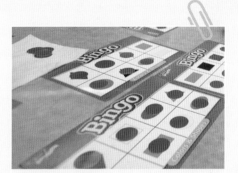

Shapes bingo
These cards have shapes instead of numbers. Match the colors or shapes to win.

Board game challenge

Playing a board game provides an opportunity to relax, talk, and laugh together. Try something new or enjoy old family favorites.

How to do it

Choose a game that is hard enough to challenge you, but not so difficult that it is frustrating.

■ It is best to play board games in teams, so you can draw on a range of skills and abilities between you.

■ To avoid stress, increase the time limit for completing a game task, set a limit to overall playing time, or build in a coffee break.

■ The main aim of any board game is to enjoy it, not to win it.

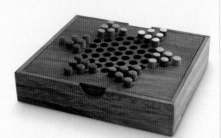

▲ Games can be simplified by reducing the number of squares or pieces.

HOW IT HELPS

Playing board games stimulates many different parts of the brain to work together creatively and logically, which may help with cognitive function.

• Many games are thought-provoking and require attention, concentration, planning, turn taking, and memory recall.

• Fine motor skills are used to manipulate game pieces.

• Games are social activities, so they can alleviate stress and depression, which in turn may support memory and cognitive function.

TALK ABOUT...

Which games were your family favorites?

•

Describe some traditional board games

•

"It is not the winning, it is the taking part" ... do you agree?

Would you describe yourself as competitive?

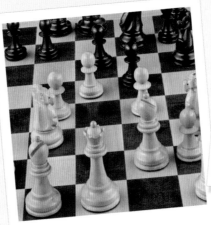

Chess

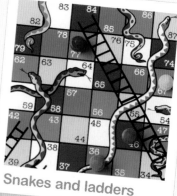

Snakes and ladders

▶ Board games challenge memory, drawing ability, reasoning, and word or numerical skills, depending on which one you choose.

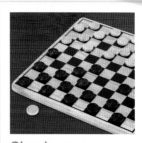

Checkers

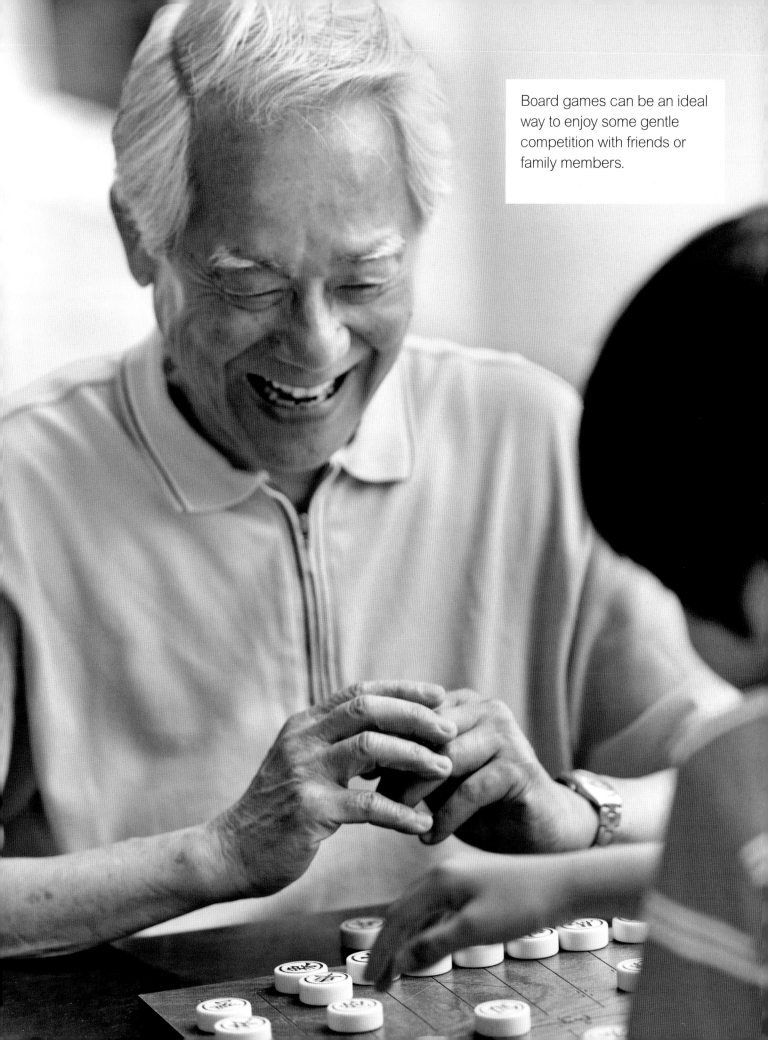

Board games can be an ideal way to enjoy some gentle competition with friends or family members.

The Seven Wonders of the World

In ancient times, great thinkers and scholars had described seven architectural wonders of the world. Unfortunately, only one of those original landmarks—the Great Pyramids—still exists. So, in 2007, the seven wonders of the modern world were chosen by popular vote in a worldwide poll. They are illustrated here.

Can you think of any other man-made marvels that could have been considered for the list?

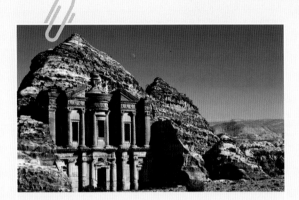

Petra
Also known as the Rose City, this ancient city in Jordan has many ornate tombs and temples carved into the pink sandstone cliffs.

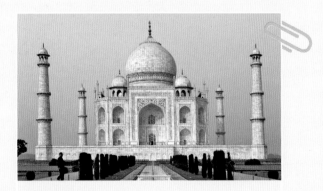

Taj Mahal
This beautiful building, in Agra, India, was built by the Mughal emperor Shah Jahan in honor of Mumtaz Mahal, his beloved third wife.

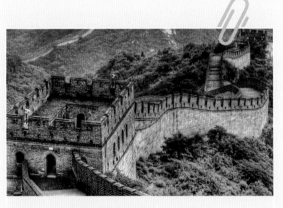

Great Wall of China
Built between the 5th century CE and the 16th century, this is the longest man-made structure, spanning 4,000 miles (6,440 km).

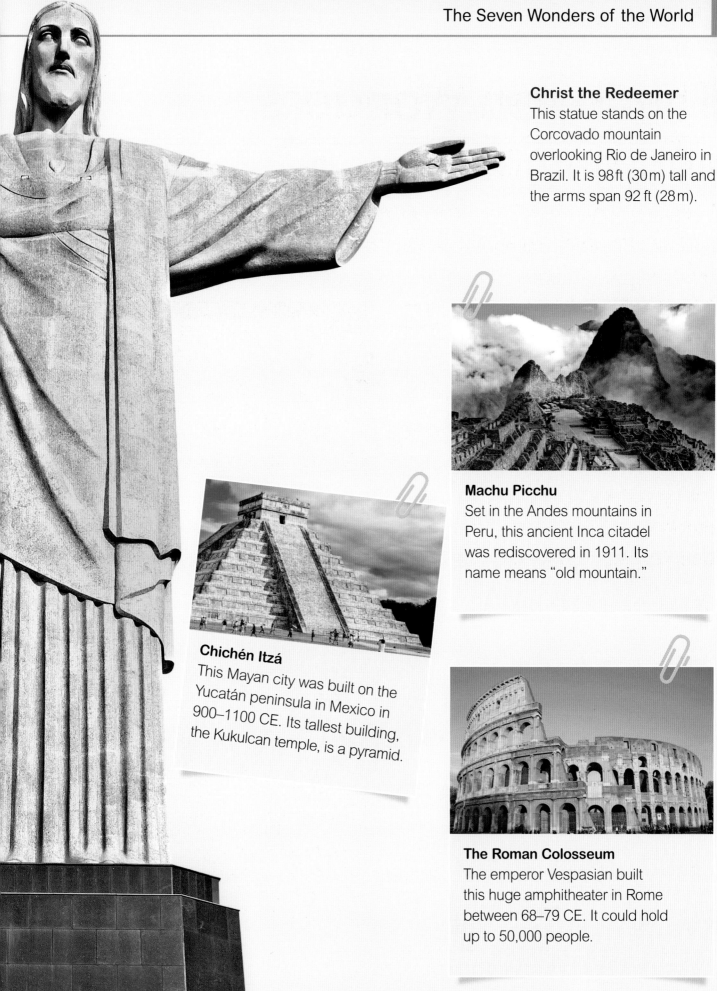

Christ the Redeemer
This statue stands on the Corcovado mountain overlooking Rio de Janeiro in Brazil. It is 98 ft (30 m) tall and the arms span 92 ft (28 m).

Machu Picchu
Set in the Andes mountains in Peru, this ancient Inca citadel was rediscovered in 1911. Its name means "old mountain."

Chichén Itzá
This Mayan city was built on the Yucatán peninsula in Mexico in 900–1100 CE. Its tallest building, the Kukulcan temple, is a pyramid.

The Roman Colosseum
The emperor Vespasian built this huge amphitheater in Rome between 68–79 CE. It could hold up to 50,000 people.

Pattern puzzles and games

There is a huge range of pattern puzzles available. Try different ones—on your own or with family and friends. The important thing is to have fun.

How to do it

Choose a pattern puzzle that suits your strengths and experience. For example, if you have always enjoyed dominoes, you may find it easier and more enjoyable than if you are new to the game.

■ You may find it helpful to create a memory card (see pages 204–205) to help remind you of the rules of a particular game.

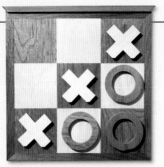

▲ Tic-tac-toe is a strategy game that can be played with one other player.

AT A GLANCE
✓ Sedentary
✓ 1 or more people
✓ Self-care/leisure
✓ Variable timeframe
✓ Variable difficulty

HOW IT HELPS

Enjoying a puzzle releases endorphins (feel-good hormones) into the body, increasing your well-being and reducing stress and anxiety, which in turn lowers blood pressure.

• Solving puzzles uses cognitive skills such as short-term memory, concentration, reasoning, decision-making, and problem-solving.

• Visual perception and spatial processing are needed to recognize patterns.

• Manipulating pieces of a game practices hand-eye coordination, visuospatial awareness, and fine motor skills.

• Procedural memory is involved in completing familiar puzzles and games.

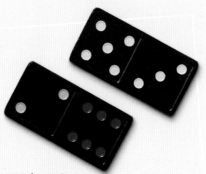

Dominoes
The patterns are easier to see if the dots contrast in color with the dominoes.

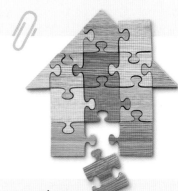

Larger sizes
If your eyesight is failing, look for puzzles or playing pieces in larger sizes.

TALK ABOUT...

Other pattern puzzle games that you like

•

Did you play marbles as a child?

•

Puzzles that you could enjoy with younger members of the family

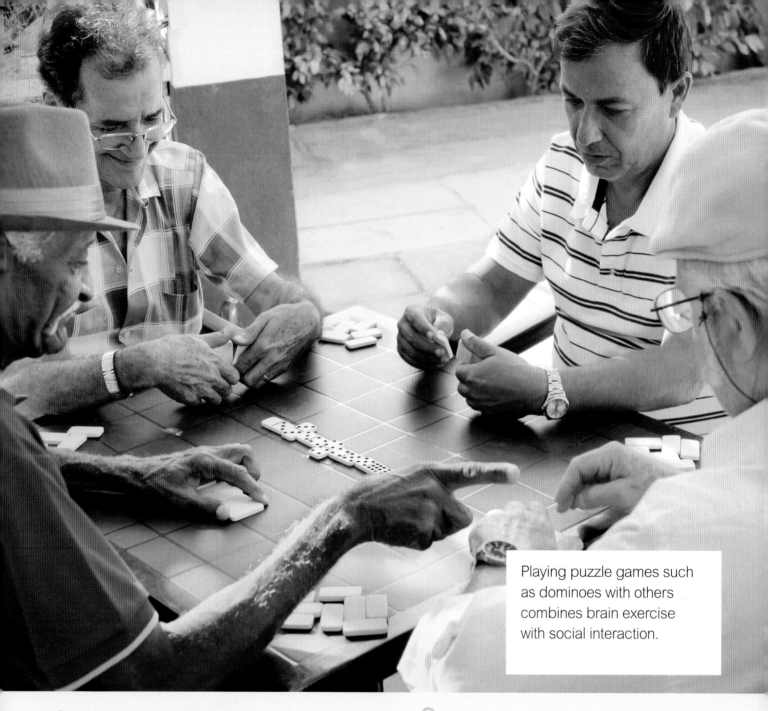

Playing puzzle games such as dominoes with others combines brain exercise with social interaction.

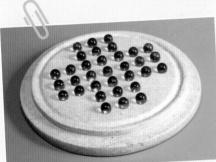

Marble solitaire
You play this board puzzle on your own. It is easy to leave and come back to later.

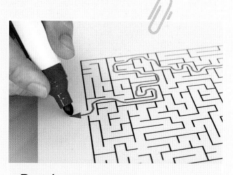

Puzzles on paper
You could enlarge paper puzzles on a photocopier to make them easier to see.

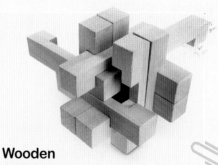

Wooden 3-D puzzles
Most 3-D puzzles are complex but, even if you can't solve them, are soothing to handle.

Play a card game

If you enjoy playing cards, simple adaptations can help you to continue to play your favorite games, or you could try a new game.

How to do it

Find a card game that is just challenging enough for you to enjoy playing. You do not need to struggle with a complex game.

■ Try variations of favorite games. For example: each player turns over a card and whoever has the highest number wins the pair.

■ Lay a small number of cards face down. Lift one card and guess the position of its match. If it matches, remove the pair. Continue until all cards are used.

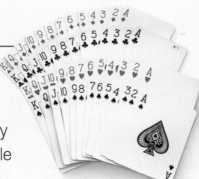

▲ If you prefer a simpler card game, sort a deck of cards into suits or by number, and use half a pack instead.

AT A GLANCE

✓ Sedentary

✓ 1 or more people

✓ Leisure

✓ Variable timeframe

✓ Variable difficulty

! Beware of games involving money stakes or gambling

HOW IT HELPS

Playing cards involves cognitive skills of concentration, attention, decision-making, problem solving, mental arithmetic, and reasoning.

• Card games rehearse recognition of colors, shapes, and numbers.

• Many card games require quick recall, which helps to retain working memory and slow its decline.

• Manipulating cards exercises a range of fine motor skills and hand-eye coordination.

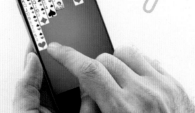

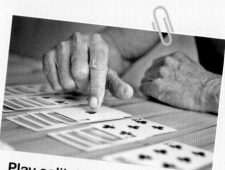

Large playing cards
If you have dexterity or vision problems, extra-large playing cards are easier to handle and see; order them online.

Online card games
Electronic versions of card games are available as apps to download to your tablet, smartphone, or computer.

Play solitaire
Solitaire is a moderately complex game that you can play on your own to practice number recognition.

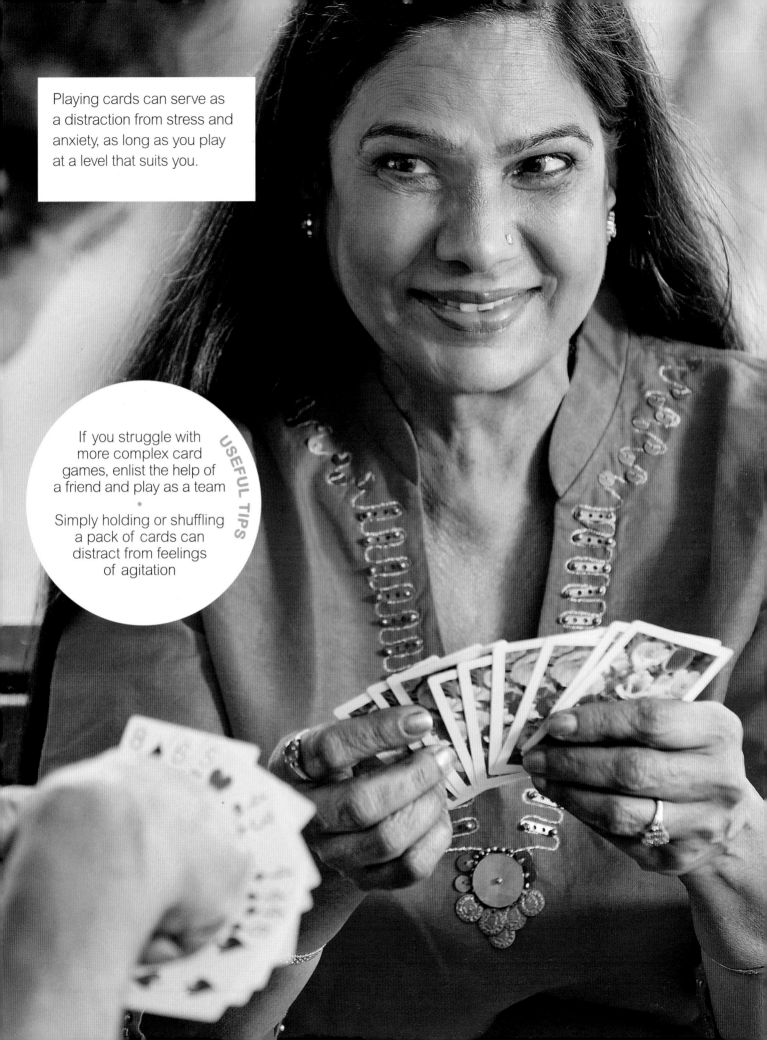

Playing cards can serve as a distraction from stress and anxiety, as long as you play at a level that suits you.

If you struggle with more complex card games, enlist the help of a friend and play as a team

Simply holding or shuffling a pack of cards can distract from feelings of agitation

Play a picture-card game

If you find standard playing cards too challenging, you can still enjoy a game of cards using picture cards. You could even make your own cards.

How to do it

Decide which game you want to play and assemble your cards. You may choose to make them, buy printed cards, or download cards from a website.

■ To play Snap, two or more players each have a set of 12 similar cards. All players simultaneously turn over their cards one at a time. When two cards with the same animal turn up, the first person to shout "Snap!" wins the pile. The player who ends up with all the cards wins.

▶ Instead of animal cards for the "Guess the Animal" game shown opposite, you could use cards with a different theme.

shown opposite

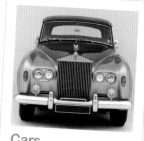

Cars

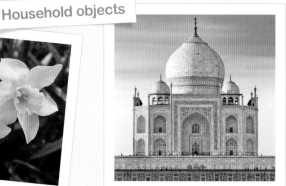

Household objects

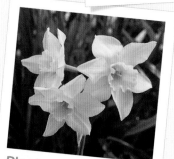

Plants

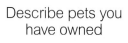

Famous landmarks

TALK ABOUT...

Describe pets you have owned
•
Which animals do you find on a farm, in a zoo, or in the ocean?
•
Name your favorite animal
•
What is the most unusual animal you have seen?

AT A GLANCE

✓ Sedentary

✓ 2 or more people

✓ Leisure

✓ 15–30 minutes

✓ Easy

! Involves use of scissors if you make your own cards

HOW IT HELPS

Playing a card game involves a range of cognitive skills, including concentration, attention, memory, and problem-solving.

• Games can be graded by limiting the number of cards or time spent playing the game. Sorting cards by categories uses a basic cognitive skill.

• Playing the game encourages communication, as well as enjoyment of gentle competition between players.

• Social elements of the game can help to improve mood and your sense of well-being.

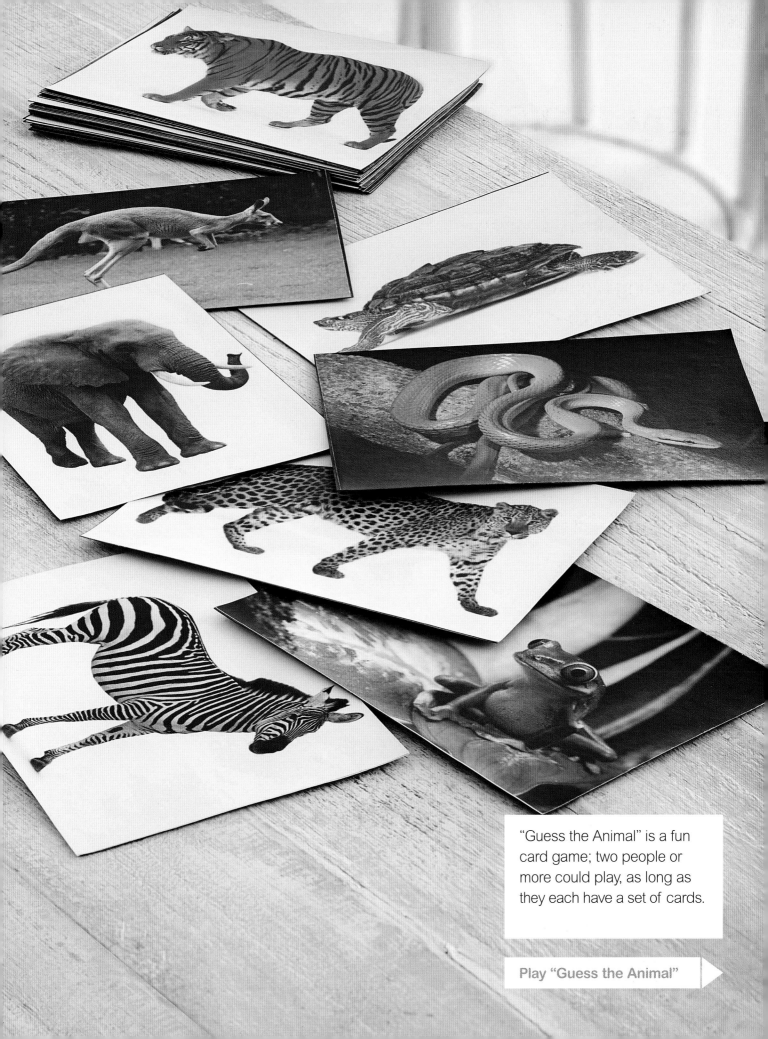

"Guess the Animal" is a fun card game; two people or more could play, as long as they each have a set of cards.

Play "Guess the Animal" ▶

Make the playing cards

When choosing pictures of animals, aim for a mix of characteristics, for example fur, hide, wool, spots, stripes, beaks, whiskers, wings, hooves, or manes. This will make the game more fun to play.

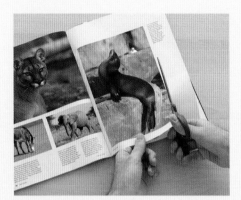

1 Look through old magazines to find 2 similar images of each animal and cut them all out. You need images for 12 animals.

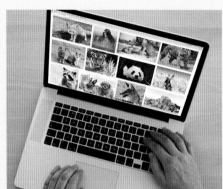

2 If you prefer, print images you have found online from the computer. Print them to 5 x 8" size.

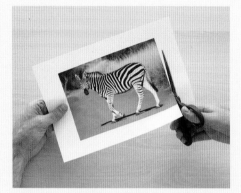

3 Cut each picture to fit one of the pieces of card. It could be the same size as the card or slightly smaller.

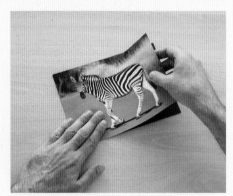

4 Spread glue over the back of each picture and glue it to a piece of card. Smooth it flat and then put aside to dry.

▶ Once dry, the cards are ready for the game. If you wish, you could outline the cards with thick black pen to make them clearer.

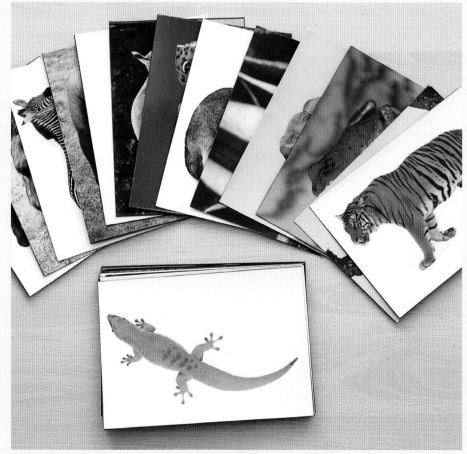

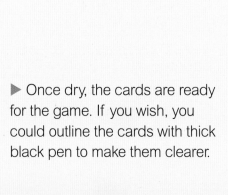

Play "Guess the Animal"

This game eliminates cards to guess the animal. Having more than 12 animal cards for each set makes the game more difficult. If you have extra sets of 12 cards, more people can play the game.

WHAT YOU NEED

Two sets of 12 animal cards, showing similar images of 12 different animals. Here are some suggestions:

- Chimpanzee
- Dog
- Gorilla
- Cat
- Cow
- Elephant
- Lizard
- Snake
- Zebra
- Tiger
- Turtle
- Frog

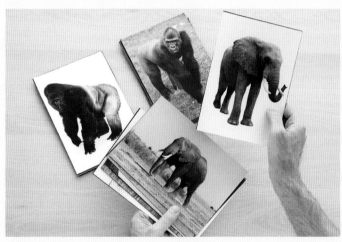

1 Sort the cards into 2 sets, so that each player has a card for every animal. Each player places his or her pile of cards picture-side down.

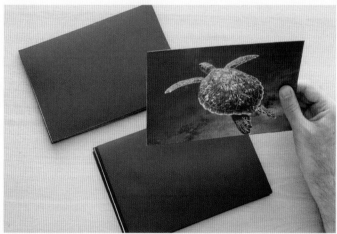

2 Player 1 chooses a card from anywhere in his or her set—that is half the pack—and keeps it hidden from the second player.

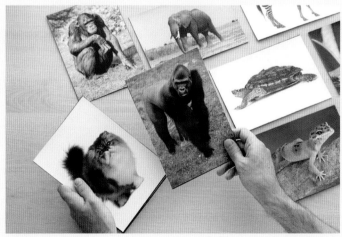

3 Player 2 lays all his or her cards face up, then asks Player 1 questions to which the answers can be "Yes" or "No." For example, "Is it furry?" If "no," all furry animals are turned over.

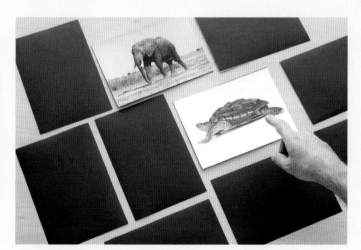

4 Continue asking relevant questions until Player 2 is left with only 1 animal. If played correctly, Player 2's last card should match that chosen by Player 1.

ARTS
AND
CRAFTS

There is a deep sense of satisfaction and achievement in making something yourself. Arts and crafts allow you to be creative and express yourself, without the need for words. Making food and baking tasty treats can be enjoyed either alone or with others (although you'll want to limit sweets). These activities often provide a form of gentle exercise, too, and stimulate your senses. Choose from a wide range of projects and ideas for creating useful, decorative, or edible items.

Painting and drawing

Whether it is your passion or you are a novice, art allows you to be creative and have fun, while benefiting your physical and mental health, and self-confidence.

How to do it

There is a style of painting or drawing to suit everyone. Experiment until you find a medium that allows you to express your creativity.

■ Prepare your materials and workspace and gather everything you will need before you start.

■ Minimizing distractions will help you to concentrate.

■ Choose nontoxic brands of oil paints, and avoid solvents such as turpentine, or switch to acrylic or poster paints.

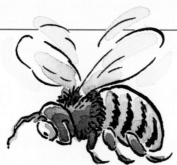

▲ The simple lines of cartoons make good images to copy. You could also photocopy them to use as coloring-in artworks.

Choosing a paintbrush
Thick-handled brushes may be easier to manage. You could also use a pierced tennis ball on the handle to improve the grip.

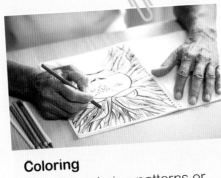

Coloring
Try adult coloring patterns or pictures. You can download images online or buy a book.

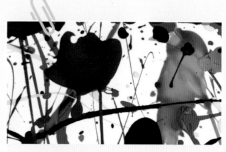

Drip painting
An abstract style frees you from pressure to produce an exact likeness. Simply drip or squirt paint on to a canvas.

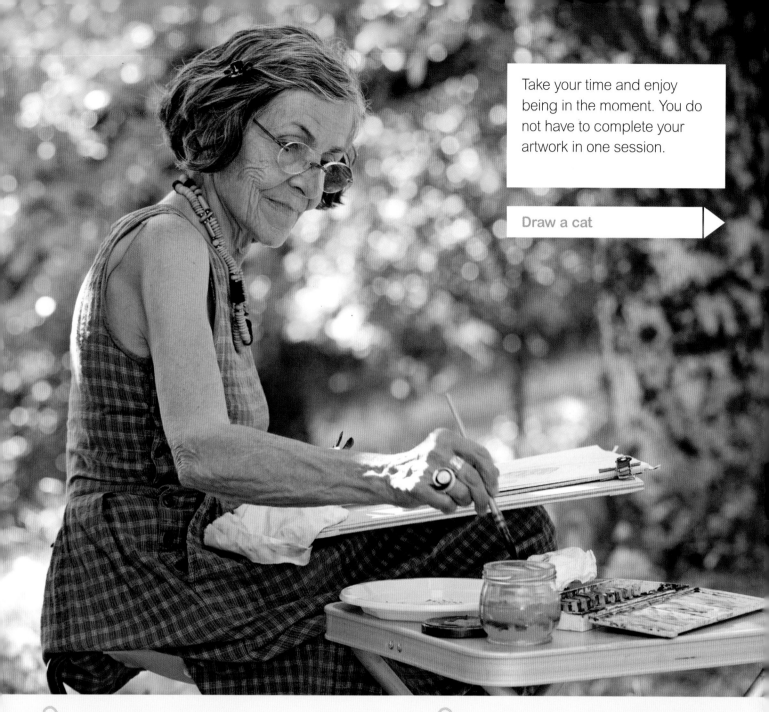

Take your time and enjoy being in the moment. You do not have to complete your artwork in one session.

Draw a cat ▷

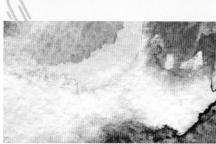

Watercolors
A simple watercolor wash can create a pleasing painting. Why not make a series, with different color combinations?

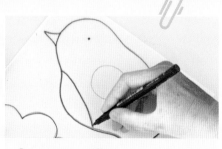

Copy an outline
If nervous about creating art, start by copying. Get help with tracing or copying lines if your eyesight makes it difficult.

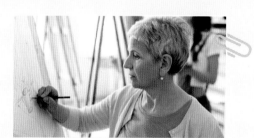

Art classes
Consider joining an art class or group so you can exchange encouragement, advice, and tips, as well as display your art.

Draw a cat

Animals might seem complicated to draw, but if you start from simple shapes and build up, it is easier than you think. It is best to use a photograph rather than drawing a live animal.

▶ Take a photograph of a pet cat, find an image in a book or magazine, or download one from the internet.

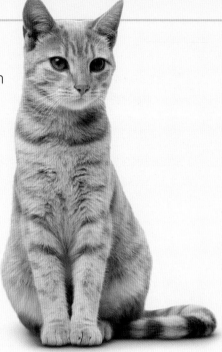

WHAT YOU NEED
- Drawing pad or paper
- Pencil
- Eraser
- Circles template (plastic stencil used in geometry—optional)
- Colored pencils or pastels

1 Draw a circle in gray pencil to denote the cat's head. Add 2 circles for the body and 3 small circles for the paws.

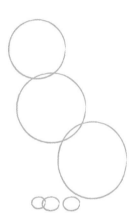

2 Using a colored pencil, join the outer edges of the 3 big circles to make the shape of the cat's body.

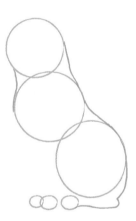

3 Draw 3 lines from the middle circle to 2 of the small circles to create the front legs.

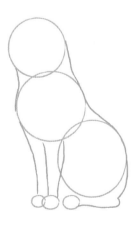

4 Add a drawing of a small circle inside the head to represent the muzzle of the cat.

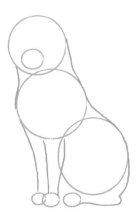

5 Trace over the head, muzzle, and paw outlines with a colored pencil. Draw in a few short lines on the paws for toes.

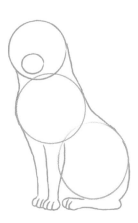

6 Draw in the cat's tail. Erase the old grey pencil lines you can still see inside the body.

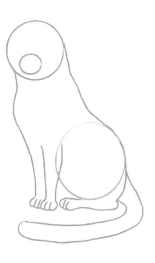

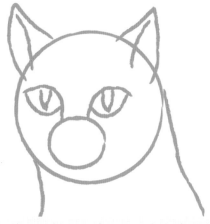

7 To sketch each ear, draw a triangle with a line down the center. Draw each eye as an oval with another oval in it.

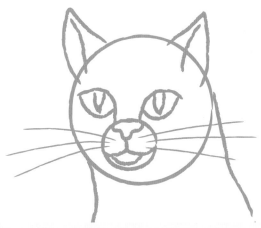

8 Draw the details of the nose on the muzzle and add a few lines for whiskers. Color in the eyes.

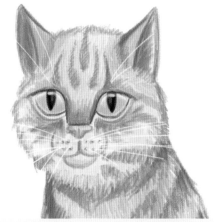

9 Draw slanting lines across the body in different shades to color in the fur.

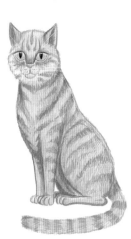

◄ This sketch is of a tabby house cat, but you could use different colors to draw other breeds of cats.

Make a pressed-flower card

The art of pressing flowers, popular in the Victorian era, captures a moment in time. Press flowers from a bouquet or your garden to serve as a reminder of a special event.

How to do it

Pressed flowers can be used in a variety of craft projects such as gift tags and other stationery, as well as the greetings card shown opposite.

▲ You could use single petals to make your own flower patterns.

■ Plan ahead and gather flowers from your garden regularly, so you have good choice of dried flowers to use.

■ Have a clean, well-lit work surface—this project involves precise work.

■ You could also make a pressed-flower picture, to bring the outdoors in, create a topic of conversation, and encourage reminiscence.

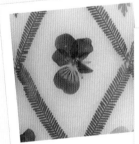

Candle

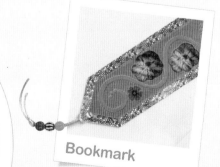

Bookmark

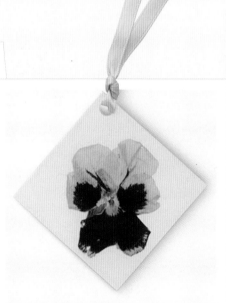

Gift tags

▲ You could use pressed flowers to decorate all sorts of items.

AT A GLANCE

✓ Sedentary

✓ 1 or 2 more people

✓ Productivity/leisure

✓ 4 weeks, then 60 minutes

! Intricate, so this is not for rheumatic fingers

! Includes use of scissors

HOW IT HELPS

Creating items with pressed flowers involves patience, concentration, and skill.

• The precise placing of delicate flowers demands a steady hand, good hand-eye coordination, and dexterity.

• Completing a challenging project such as this one can boost confidence and self-esteem.

TALK ABOUT...

What flowers do you like in posies, nosegays, and tied bunches?

•

How to use pressed flowers from a wedding bouquet or corsage

•

What else could you decorate using this technique?

▶ Use pressed flowers and foliage to decorate other types of stationery, or to create flower pictures.

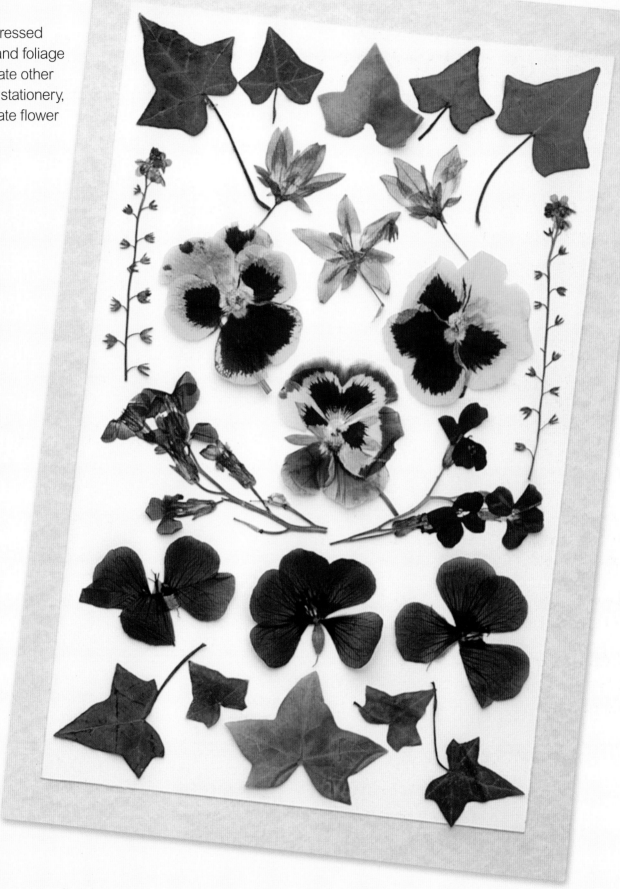

Press some flowers

Pick fresh flowers on a dry day. Flat blooms such as pansies or daisies are best. Avoid flowers with staining pollen, such as lilies. Press individual petals of bulky flowers. Don't forget to pick leaves and stems as well.

WHAT YOU NEED
- Scissors
- Blotting paper or paper towels
- Heavy books

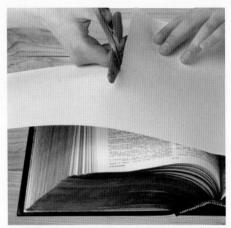

1 Open a heavy book and cut blotting paper to the size of the open pages. Fold the paper in half, then open out.

Make your pressed-flower card

Open the book pages carefully and take out the sheets of paper containing the flowers. Fold the piece of card and use the dried flowers to decorate the front of the card.

WHAT YOU NEED
- Book with pressed flowers
- Tweezers
- Toothpick
- Rubber-based glue (PVA)
- Plain card
- Scissors
- Self-stick or iron-on clear vinyl (optional)

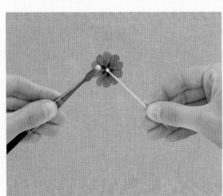

1 To stick on a flower, hold it with tweezers and apply a dab of glue to the back of it with a toothpick.

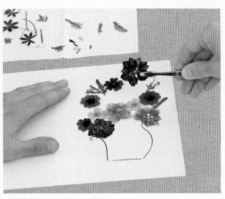

2 Use tweezers to position the flower on the card. Press down gently with the tweezers to secure the flower.

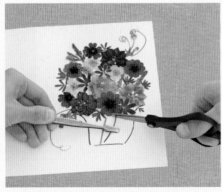

4 To add a piece of dried stem or grass, apply glue to the back. Hold it in place and then cut it to size.

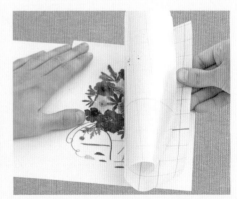

5 Leave the finished picture to dry. If you wish, seal the flowers in place with self-stick or iron-on vinyl paper.

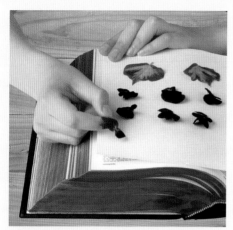

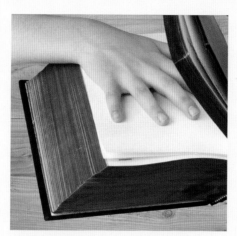

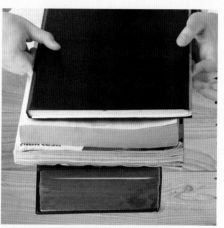

2 Space your flowers over one half page of the blotting paper. Make sure the flowers don't touch each other.

3 Fold the paper over the flowers. Hold in place as you close the book. Add more flowers between other pages.

4 Put some heavy books on top of the first one and leave to dry in a warm, dry place for about 4 weeks.

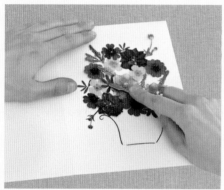

3 Stick leaves in the gaps between the flowers. Overlap some leaves with flowers to make them look realistic.

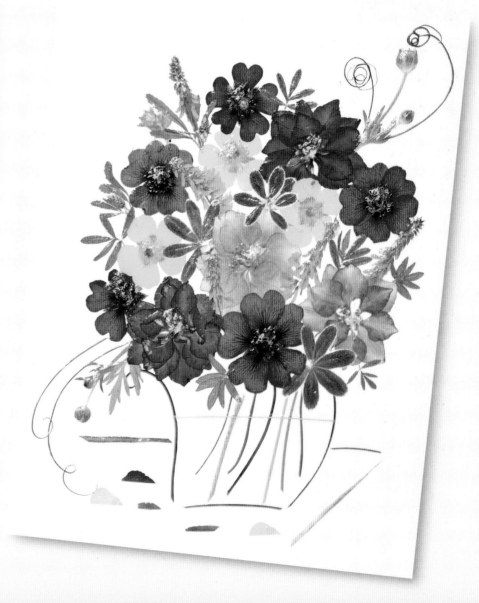

▶ This finished card has a mix of flowers and leaves in the bouquet. Grass stems have been used to "draw" a vase.

Create a collage

Even if you lack the confidence to draw or paint, you might try creating a collage. It can be as simple or as complex as you like, and it will allow you to express yourself.

How to do it

Decide on the type of collage you would like to do. Choose the collage materials: anything from old scraps of fabric or wallpaper to pages from a magazine or sheet music.

■ Protect your workspace from the glue by laying down an old cloth or newspaper.

■ Organize your collage materials by sorting them into piles of specific colors.

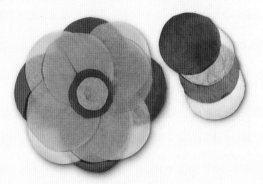

▲ Layer simple shapes to build up an image, such as circles to make up a flower.

HOW IT HELPS

This technique is a fun way to create an artwork. It stimulates the imagination, and is failure-free.

• Sorting colors and textures to create a design encourages you to plan and organize.

• Fine motor skills and hand-eye coordination is required, helping you to maintain dexterity.

• If shared with others, the process involves social interaction and communication.

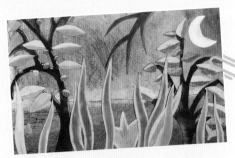

Layering a collage
Cut out parts of a picture in differently colored cards, then stick them on top of each other to create a 3-D effect.

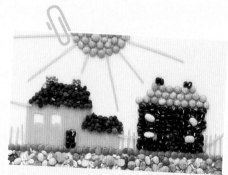

Try different materials
Use your imagination when looking for materials to use. This image was created using dry lentils, beans, and spaghetti.

TALK ABOUT...

Do you know of any famous artists who made collages?

Do you prefer making pictures or abstract patterns?

Think of other materials to use in a collage

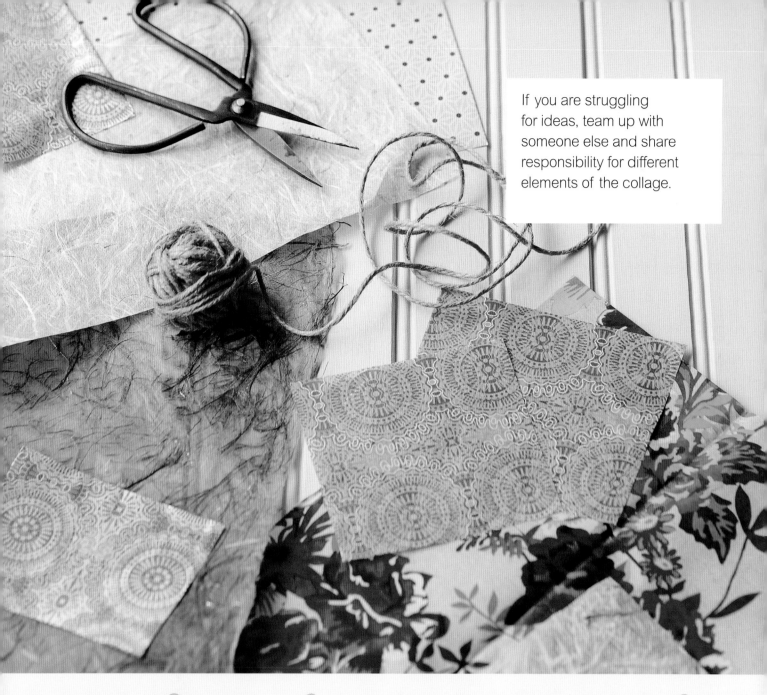

If you are struggling for ideas, team up with someone else and share responsibility for different elements of the collage.

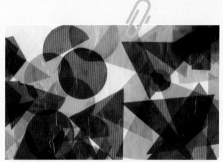

Color and shapes
Abstract patterns allow you to give free rein to your creativity without any pressure to produce a convincing likeness.

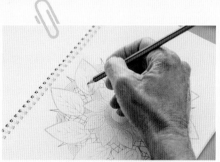

Draw a basic outline
You could draw an outline of your own image or patterns on the base and fill the outlines with different materials.

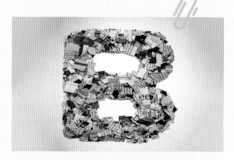

Use a ready-made image
If you are unsure of what to create, simply cover a template or a printed image with your collage materials.

Make an abstract collage

As well as the tissue paper shapes shown here, you could use larger, torn sheets of tissue paper or magazine pages to create a more layered collage. The smaller the pieces, the more intricate the end design will be and the longer it will take to complete.

WHAT YOU NEED
- Tissue paper in different colors
- Scissors
- Glue stick
- Sheet of paper or thick card

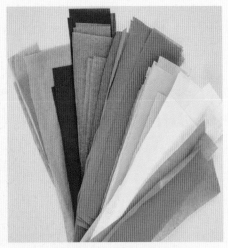

1 Collect your equipment. Choose the colors of tissue paper that you want to include in your collage.

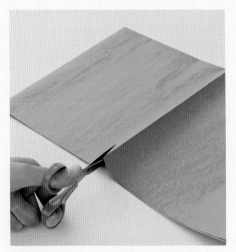

2 Cut pieces of the tissue paper into triangles of various sizes until you have about 60 individual pieces.

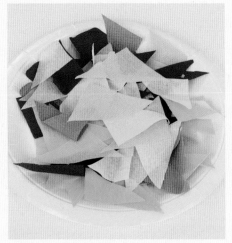

3 It helps to put the tissue paper shapes on a plate, or in a small container, so that you can use them one at a time.

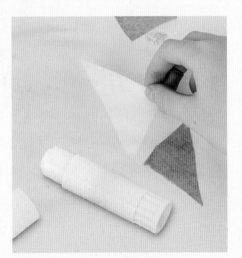

4 To paste each tissue triangle, cover one side with glue and stick it on to the paper or thick card.

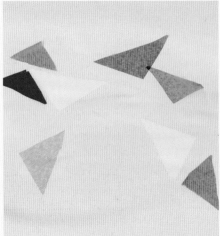

5 Smooth each piece flat to remove any air or glue bubbles. Continue sticking triangles on to the paper.

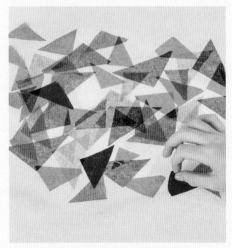

6 As you apply more pieces, overlap them so they create interlocking shapes to finish your abstract design.

Collage as decoration

You could liven up things around the home by adding colorful collages. For example, use this technique to decorate objects such as picture or photo frames, diary or scrapbook covers, greeting cards, or your memory box (see pages 88–89).

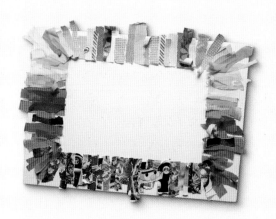

Picture frame

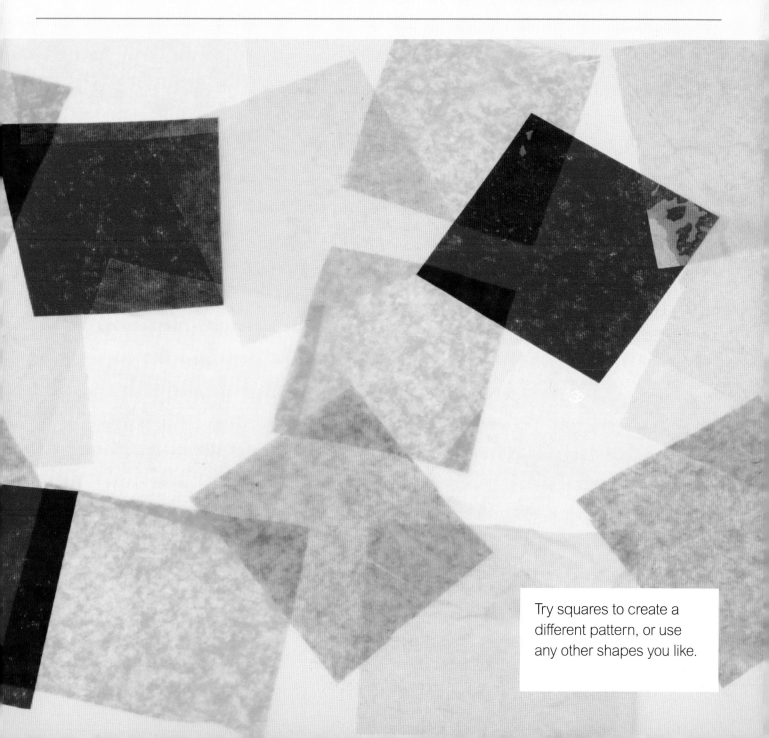

Try squares to create a different pattern, or use any other shapes you like.

Famous works of art

Human beings have been producing works of art for more than 40,000 years, and some of the earliest, cave paintings, still survive. It is now possible to see many of the best known works of art in books or online. Or perhaps you've seen some of them in museums. Easily one of the most recognizable paintings in the world is the "Mona Lisa," painted by Leonardo da Vinci, which now hangs in the Louvre in Paris.

▶ Postimpressionist artist Georges Seurat painted this large canvas, "A Sunday Afternoon on the Island of La Grande Jatte," in 1886 using the pointillist style.

Do you have a favorite painter or painting?

Which do you prefer: old masters or modern art; still lifes or abstract styles; portraits or landscapes?

Do you prefer paintings or sculptures?

TALK ABOUT...

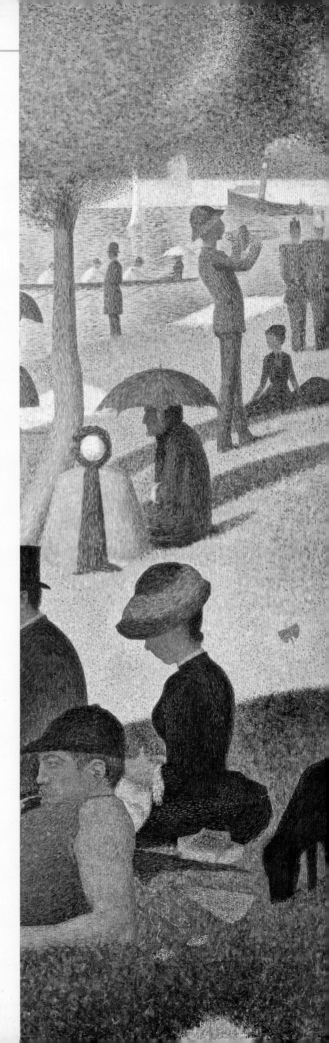

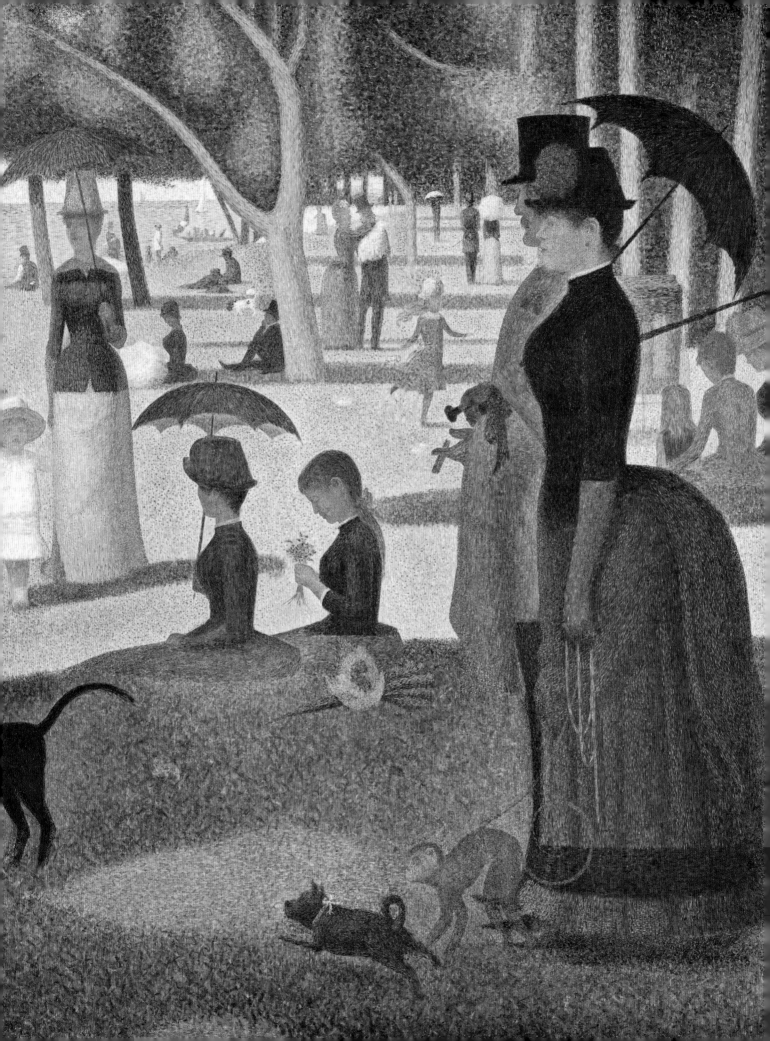

Easy printing

Printing is a lovely way of decorating plain items of clothing and creating artwork, greetings cards, and wrapping papers.

How to do it

Cover your workspace with an old cloth and wear an apron or old clothes—printing can get messy—and gather everything you need to create your print.

■ Apply paint or ink to your stamp with a small roller, or place the stamp on an inkpad or in a shallow dish of paint.

■ Press the stamp evenly on to card, fabric, or a canvas to create your print.

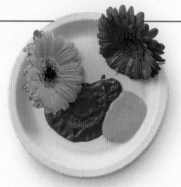

▲ Look for things around you to use as printing stamps—flat flower heads make good stamps.

HOW IT HELPS

Creative arts, such as printing, can boost confidence and self-esteem and offer a way of expressing yourself when words become difficult.

• Printing is fun, simple, and failure-free.

• The immediate nature of printing could help to motivate you to do more.

• All stages of this technique require concentration, good hand-eye coordination, and a steady hand.

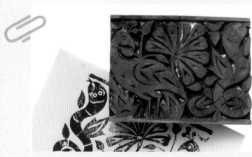

Linocut block
If you are unsure about creating a design, you could use a printing block with a ready-made linocut design on it.

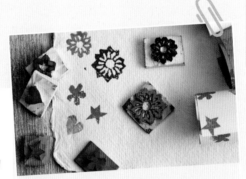

Ready-made stamp
You could choose from a huge range of ready-made stamps and stencils available in craft stores and online.

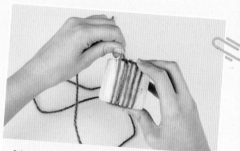

Homemade stamp
Glue string around a wood block for a geometric pattern; hold at different angles to print with it.

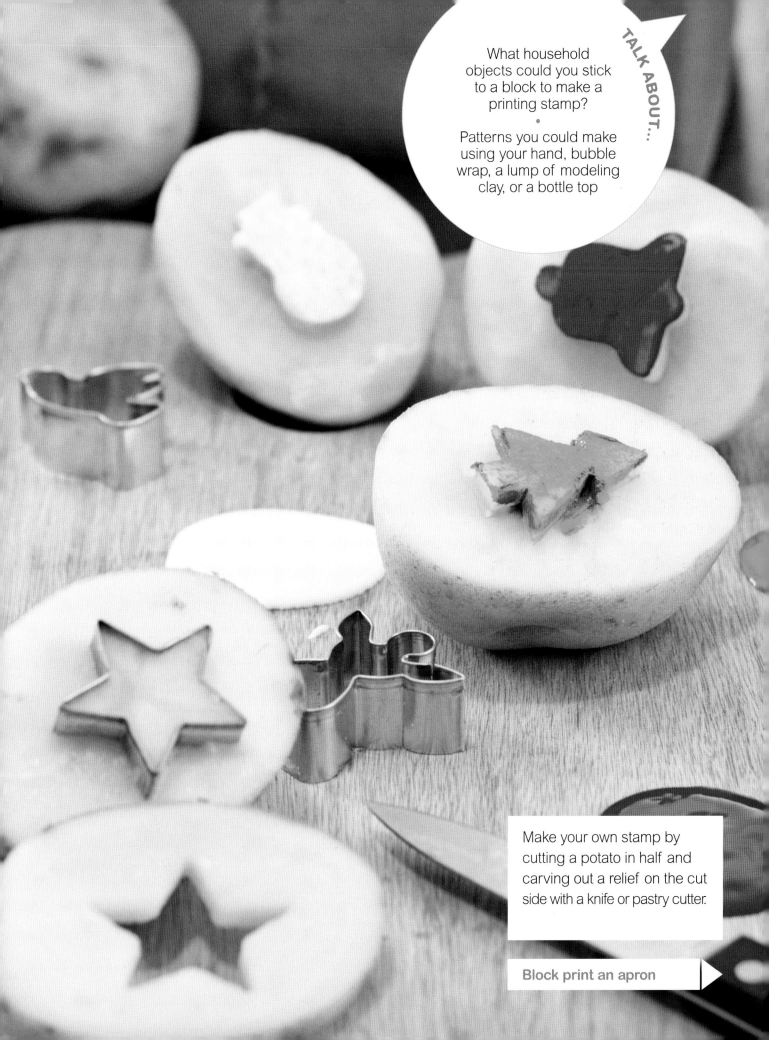

TALK ABOUT...

What household objects could you stick to a block to make a printing stamp?

Patterns you could make using your hand, bubble wrap, a lump of modeling clay, or a bottle top

Make your own stamp by cutting a potato in half and carving out a relief on the cut side with a knife or pastry cutter.

Block print an apron ▶

Create templates for your design

Use these fish and citrus motifs by copying the shapes onto paper, or enlarge them on a photocopier and trace them to make templates. Alternatively, you could be creative and make your own designs. You may want to prepare the block stamps and do the printing on separate occasions to avoid getting tired.

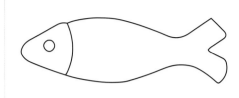
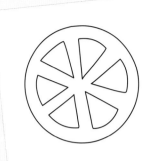

Fish

Citrus slice

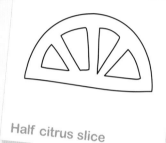

Half citrus slice

▲ Use a thick, black pen to draw or trace these designs onto paper.

Block print an apron

Most dyes need to be "fixed" into place by ironing, so check the manufacturer's instructions on the paints before you use them. Ask for help with the more complex steps, if they are too challenging.

WHAT YOU NEED
- Plain cotton or linen apron
- Paper templates
- Scissors
- Sheet of craft foam
- Pencil
- All-purpose glue
- 3 small wooden blocks
- Medium-sized paintbrush
- Fabric paints in 3 different colors
- Clean cloth or paper
- Iron

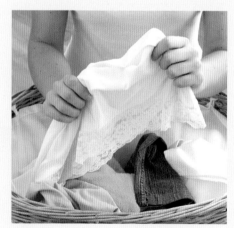

1 Wash your apron before printing on it: many fabric paints work best on freshly laundered items. Cotton or linen fabrics often work best.

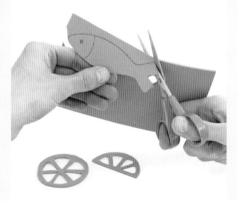

2 Cut out each paper template. Place on a piece of craft foam. Draw around each template. Cut out a matching foam shape.

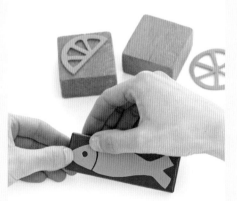

3 Glue each foam shape to a block. Cut the fish's head off the template. Leave a thin gap between the body and head when gluing them in place.

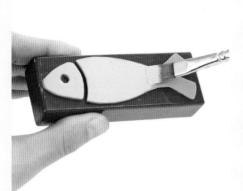

4 Use the paintbrush to apply a thin, even layer of blue fabric paint to the foam shape of the fish block.

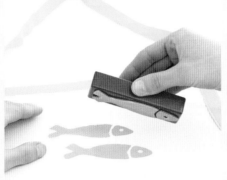

5 Press the paint-covered block on the apron to print the fish. Reapply paint to the block each time you want to make a print.

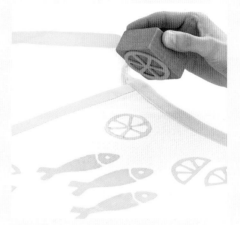

6 Repeat the process with yellow and green paint to print some citrus motifs. Leave the printed apron to dry completely.

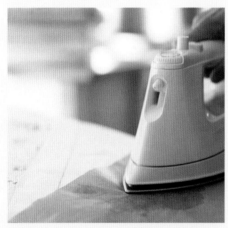

7 If necessary, set the paints by placing a clean cloth or paper over the printed area and ironing it with a hot iron.

▶ Why not decorate other kitchen linens to match? You could print oven gloves or dish towels, for example.

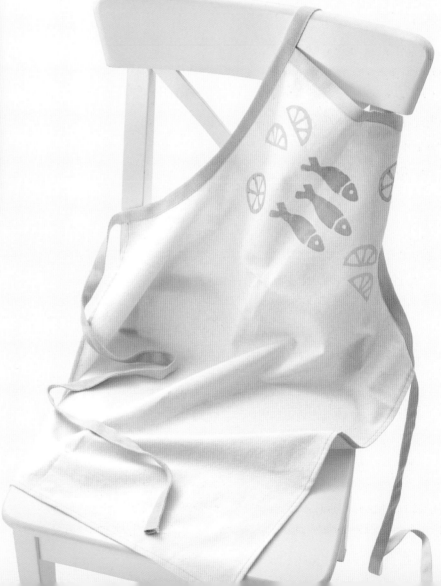

Make a papier-mâché bowl

This easy technique allows you to be creative, is failure-free, and is fun to share with others.

How to do it

Decide how you are going to use the bowl. Do you want it for holding jewelry, your keys, or some potpourri? Or perhaps to display sweets, fruit, or shells? This will dictate the size.

■ Prepare your work surface by covering it with old newspapers or a wipeable cloth. Find everything you need in advance.

■ Once you have made the bowl, you can be as creative as you like when you decorate it. If it is for a child, you may choose bright colors. If it is for yourself, you could paint it in your favorite color.

▶ Finish the papier-mâché bowl with layers of colored tissue paper or strips from a colorful comic, or paint it once it is dry.

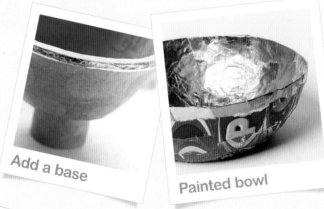
Add a base

Painted bowl

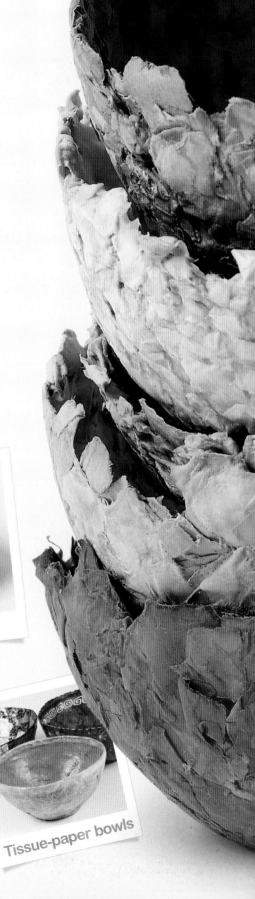

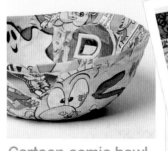
Cartoon-comic bowl

Tissue-paper bowls

TALK ABOUT...

Papier-mâché means "chewed paper" in French.

What else do you use old newspapers for?

Other things you could make from papier-mâché

Do you have anything made in papier-mâché in your home?

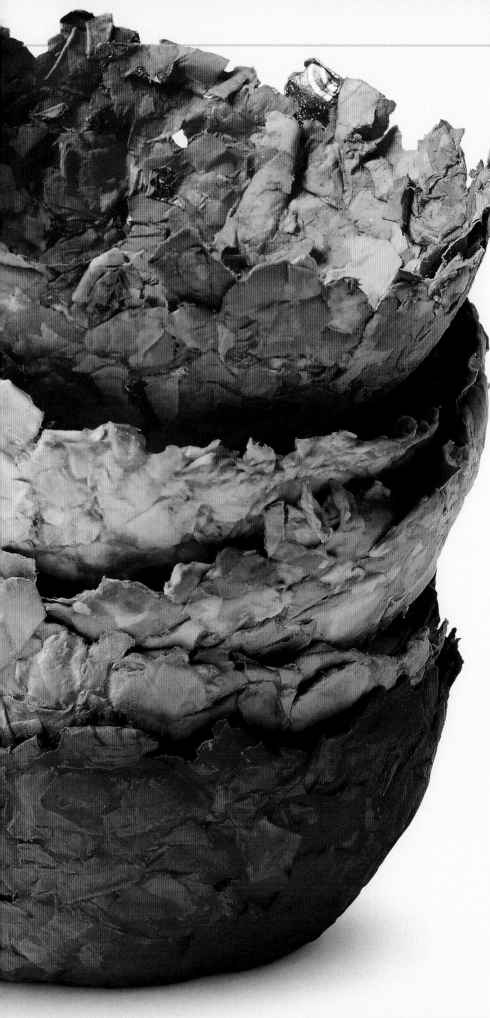

AT A GLANCE

✓ Sedentary

✓ 1 or more people

✓ Productivity

✓ 30 minutes for each step, plus drying time

✓ Easy

! Involves use of stovetop or wallpaper paste with fungicide, and scissors

HOW IT HELPS

This project can be done in stages over a number of days if your concentration is limited.

• Tearing the paper is relaxing and uses fine finger movements, exercising your dexterity.

• Layering the papier-mâché helps to maintain hand-eye coordination.

• This project needs planning and organizational skills; sequencing through the activity also exercises and helps to maintain cognitive skills.

◀ If you use the same mold, you could make a set of bowls in contrasting colors.

Collect some paper

Old newspapers are best because the paper is porous and soaks up the paste easily, but you will need to paint it once it is dry. You could use colored paper, such as old gift wrap or tissue paper, to give the bowl its basic color.

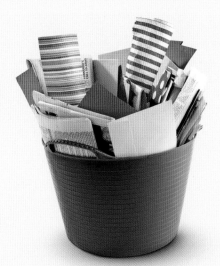

Colored paper

WHAT YOU NEED

- Old newspapers
- 3 cups water, divided
- 1 cup flour
- Saucepan
- Wooden spoon
- Bowl or glass jar
- Plastic bowl (for the mold)
- Petroleum jelly
- Paintbrush
- Scissors
- Rubber gloves (optional)
- Food-safe paint (optional)

Make a papier-mâché bowl

This is made with a flour and water paste that needs to be used fresh. To make the bowl in stages, mix wallpaper paste and keep it in a jar with a lid to use again. Wallpaper paste contains fungicide, so wash your hands or wear rubber gloves.

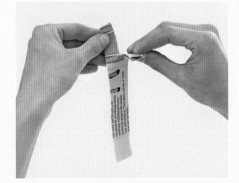

1 Tear the paper into strips that are roughly the same width as the bowl. They don't have to be exactly the same size.

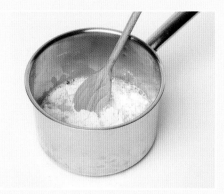

2 Put 1 cup of water and the flour into the saucepan. Heat gently and stir the mixture until it is a smooth paste.

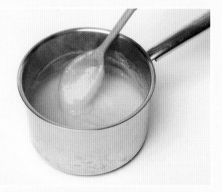

3 Add the remaining 2 cups of water. Bring to a boil, stirring constantly. Pour into a bowl or jar and allow to cool.

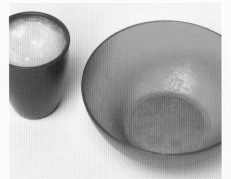

4 Grease the plastic bowl you are using as a mold with petroleum jelly to prevent the paper from sticking to the bowl.

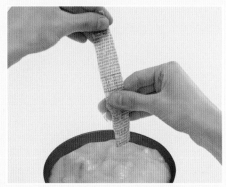

5 Take a paper strip and dip it into the paste so it is soaked completely. Wipe off surplus paste with your fingers.

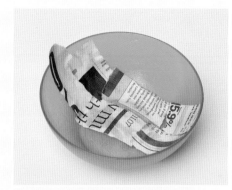

6 Lay the strip across the inside of the bowl. Soak another strip in paste. Lay it in the bowl so it overlaps the first strip.

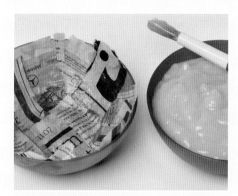

7 Continue until the bowl is covered in paper past the edges. Brush the entire layer with more paste.

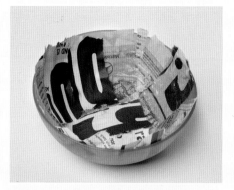

8 Add more strips of soaked paper across the bowl to build up another layer of paper. Keep overlapping the strips.

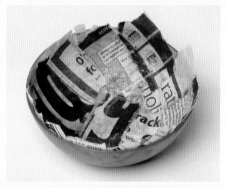

9 Brush another coat of paste over the second layer of paper. Keep adding layers of paper until you have 6 layers.

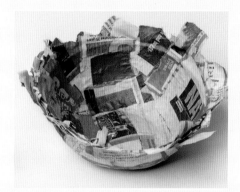

10 Leave the bowl overnight to dry completely. Discard any leftover paste; it should wash away under running water.

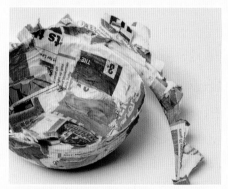

11 Gently remove the bowl from its mold. Trim the edge with scissors. Your bowl is ready to decorate and paint.

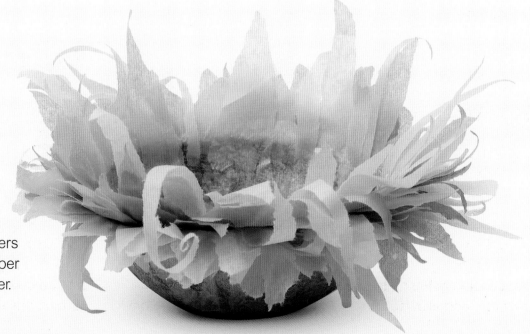

▶ This bowl was made with 10–12 layers of colored tissue paper instead of newspaper.

Working with wood

A woodworking project can be deeply satisfying on a sensory level and give you a sense of achievement. You could make something from scratch or from precut wood.

How to do it

Choose a project to complete that suits your experience and current level of woodworking skills.

▪ If you prefer to sit at a table, try sanding precut wooden kit pieces and assembling, painting, or varnishing them.

▪ A long-term project, such as refurbishing an old piece of furniture, involves a variety of tasks and you can return to it whenever you want.

▪ Consider joining a local woodworking club. It offers a chance to chat, reminisce, and support each other.

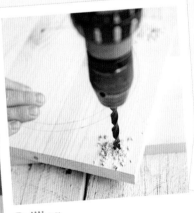

Drilling

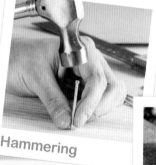

Hammering

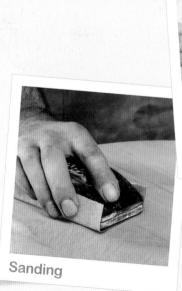

Sanding

▲ You may prefer to use your experience and woodworking skills by helping with familiar tasks in a shared project.

Sawing

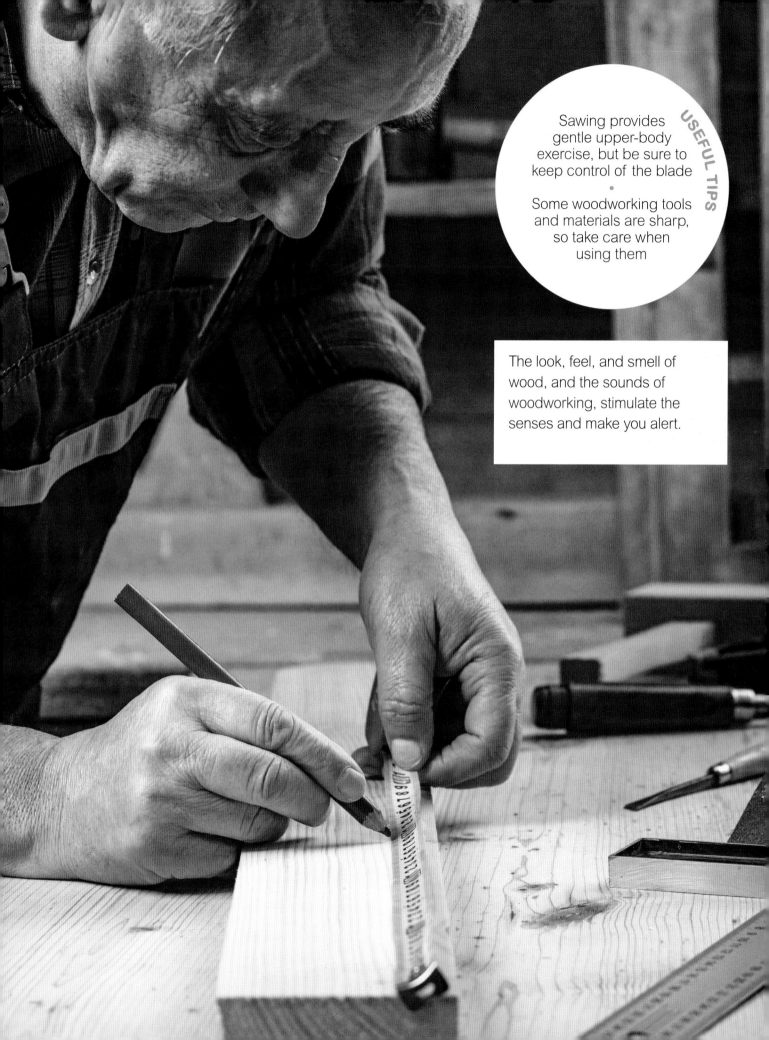

USEFUL TIPS

Sawing provides gentle upper-body exercise, but be sure to keep control of the blade

Some woodworking tools and materials are sharp, so take care when using them

The look, feel, and smell of wood, and the sounds of woodworking, stimulate the senses and make you alert.

Make a window box

A planter is relatively easy to make with some basic tools and one plank of wood, especially if you have experience in DIY.

How to do it

Concentrate on the steps that you feel confident about, whether it is sawing or simply sharing words of wisdom.

■ Use this project as an opportunity to share your expertise with younger family members.

■ If you find dealing with measurements challenging, you could buy a kit, with pieces already cut to size, and assemble it.

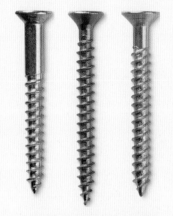

▲ Make sure that you use wood screws of the correct length.

HOW IT HELPS

If you enjoy working with wood, simple projects such as this will maintain your skills.

• Rehearsing an old skill engages procedural memory, gives you a sense of achievement, and improves your confidence and self-esteem.

• This project demands a range of cognitive skills, including planning, organizing, following sequences, concentrating, and problem-solving.

• Using tools involves hand-eye coordination and strength.

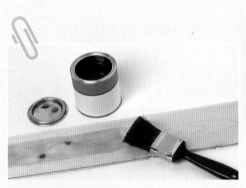

Wood paint
You could use a water-based, nontoxic wood stain to color the window box. Paint it before adding any slug tape.

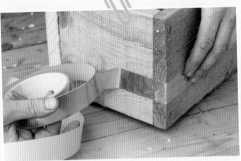

Slug tape
To stop slugs from munching the plants, press and tack copper adhesive tape around the lower part of the window box.

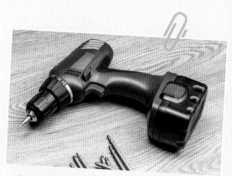

Power tools
If unsure about using power tools, get help with difficult steps such as drilling.

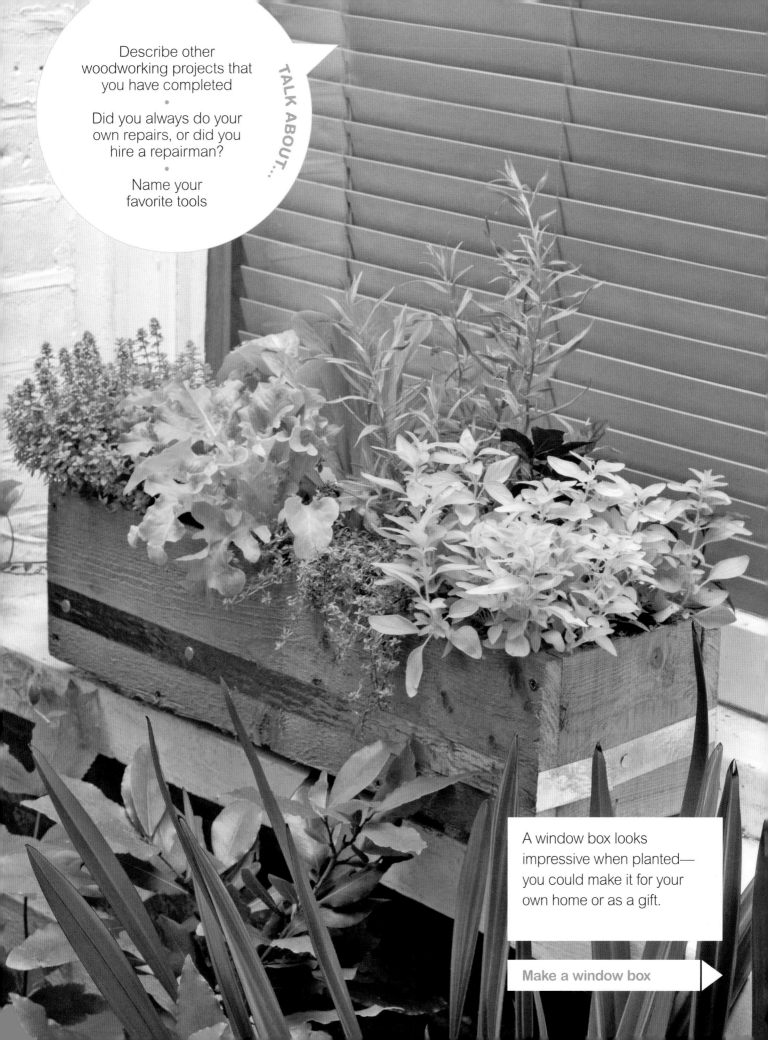

TALK ABOUT…

Describe other woodworking projects that you have completed

Did you always do your own repairs, or did you hire a repairman?

Name your favorite tools

A window box looks impressive when planted— you could make it for your own home or as a gift.

Make a window box ▶

Measuring the pieces

Choose a 1 in (2.5 cm) thick plank that is long enough to cut out all the window box pieces. You may have to trim a longer plank down to 82 in (205 cm). Here is a guide on how to measure the plank when you mark it up for sawing.

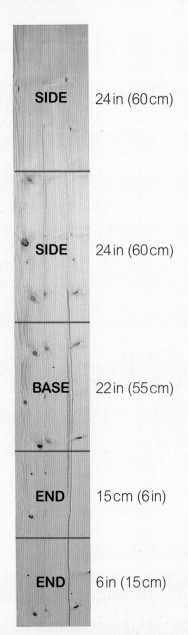

SIDE	24 in (60 cm)
SIDE	24 in (60 cm)
BASE	22 in (55 cm)
END	15 cm (6 in)
END	6 in (15 cm)

Make a window box

When measuring the plank, use the diagram shown to the left as a guide. Double-check that you have measured correctly. Draw a line straight across the plank at right angles to each measured point—you might find it easier to do this if you use a T-square. Alternatively, you could measure the pieces from separate scraps of wood, but make sure they are all 1 in (2.5 cm) thick.

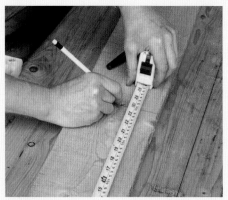

1 On the plank, measure where to cut out the 2 sides, base, and 2 ends. Draw pencil lines to mark it out.

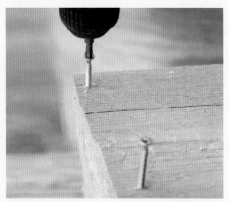

5 Use 2 screws to align both pilot holes with those in the end piece. Finish screwing in the screws with the screwdriver.

WHAT YOU NEED

- 1 plank or pressure-treated board: 6 x 1 x 82 in (15 x 2.5 x 205 cm)
- Pencil
- Ruler
- Measuring tape
- Wood saw
- 20 self-tapping, 2 in (50 mm) long wood screws

- 4 self-tapping, 1½ in (38 mm) long wood screws (for battens)
- Rechargeable screwdriver
- Drill and drill bits
- 2 battens: 1 x ½ x 7 in (25 x 12 x 180 mm)
- T-square (optional)

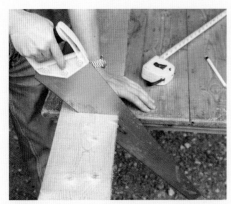

2 Saw the plank into pieces, following your markings. For a neat cut, get a helper to hold the other end of the plank.

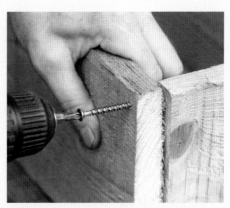

3 Attach an end piece to a side piece, at the 2 corners of the side piece. You could screw directly into the wood.

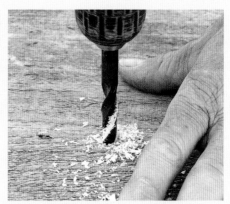

4 Alternatively, it might be easier if you drill pilot holes first. Use a drill bit that is one size smaller than the screws.

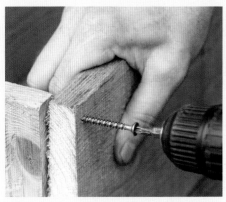

6 Repeat steps 3 to 5 to attach the second end piece to the side piece. You now have a 3-sided frame; place it on its side.

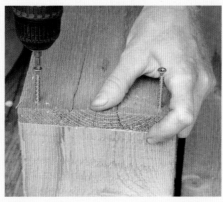

7 Lay the second side piece on top so that its edges line up with the end pieces. Screw it to the end pieces at its 4 corners.

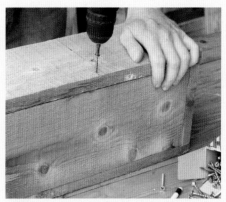

8 Place the base piece into the 4-sided frame. If it doesn't fit, mark where to cut against the frame and trim it.

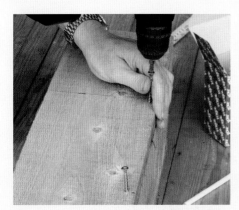

9 Fix the base in position by inserting screws through pilot holes on both sides. Space them about 6 in (15 cm) apart.

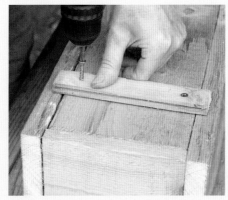

10 Turn the box upside down. Set the 2 battens on the base, 1 at each end. Attach each batten with 2 screws.

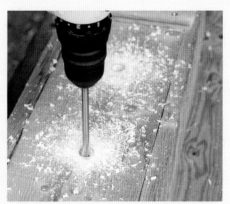

11 Drill some drainage holes in the base. Space the holes about 4 in (10 cm) apart. Don't drill into the work surface!

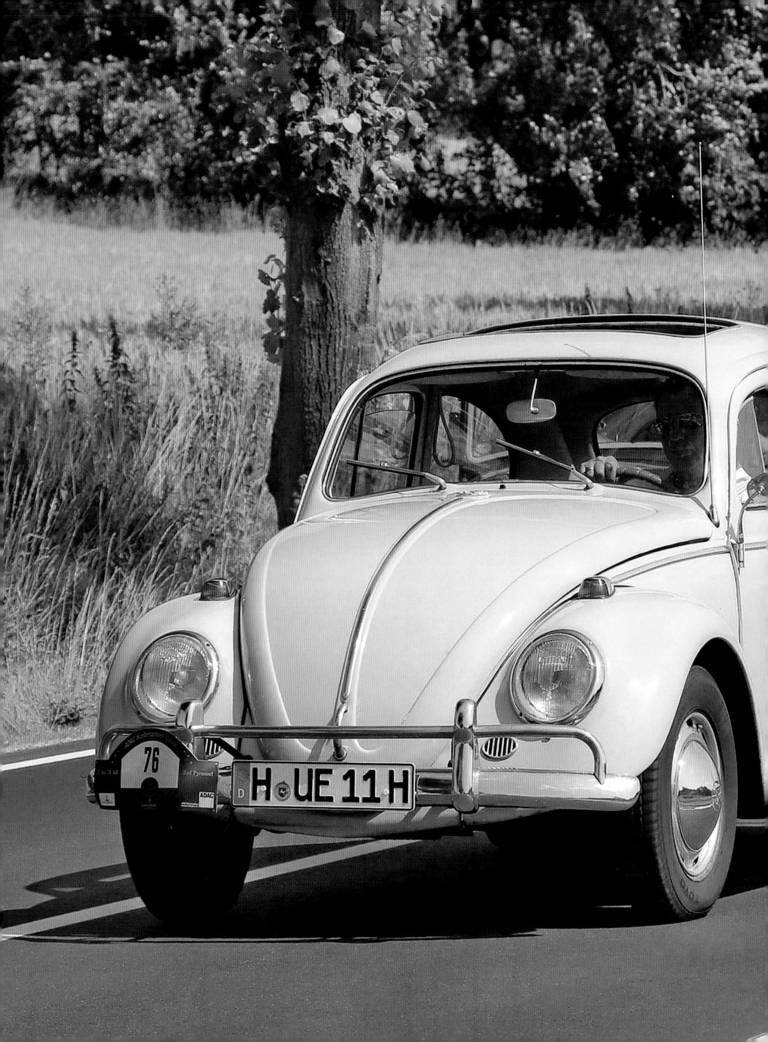

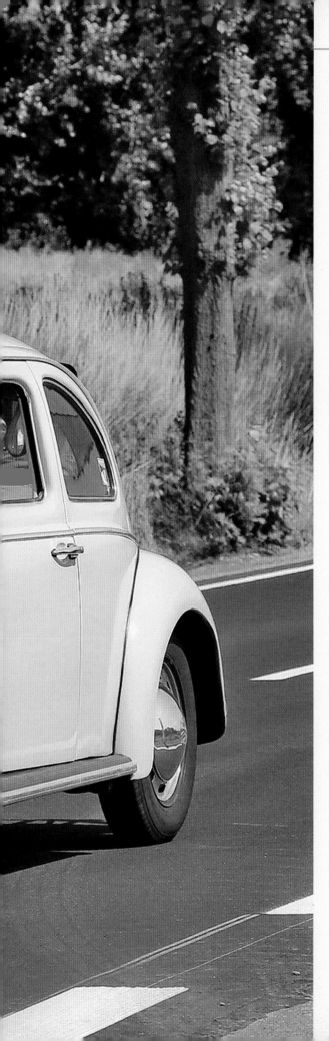

Classic cars

The Ford Model T brought ownership of a car within reach of the ordinary person more than a century ago. Since then, some car designs have caught the imagination of car enthusiasts and become classics. Makes such as Rolls-Royce and Porsche were emblems of wealth, but others became classics through longevity. The Volkswagen Beetle, which was in production longer than any other car, is still the best-selling car of all time.

◀ Although there were different versions of the Volkswagen Beetle throughout its 65 years in production, it always retained its distinctive shape.

What was the first car you ever drove in?

What is your favorite car from film or television?

If money were no object, what dream car would you buy?

TALK ABOUT…

Bring the outdoors in

Even if you spend most of your time indoors, you can connect to the natural world by enhancing your environment with objects from nature.

How to do it

Bring the hues of the natural world into your home by painting the walls in realistic shades of green and blue.

■ Hang a painting or photograph of your favorite environment, such as a beach, mountain, or woodland scene, on the wall.

■ Fill vases with arrangements of fresh, dried, or silk flowers, grasses, and foliage.

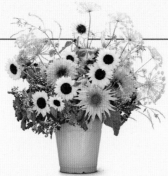

▲ Using fresh, seasonal flowers will help orientate you to the changing seasons.

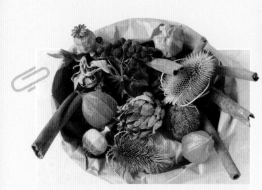

Potpourri
Make a potpourri from dried seed heads and a few drops of essential oil.

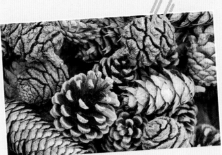

Keep a collection
Collect objects like these pine cones, and display your collection for all to see.

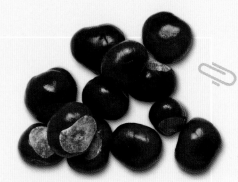

Tactile trophies
Items with different textures stimulate the senses and can be soothing to hold.

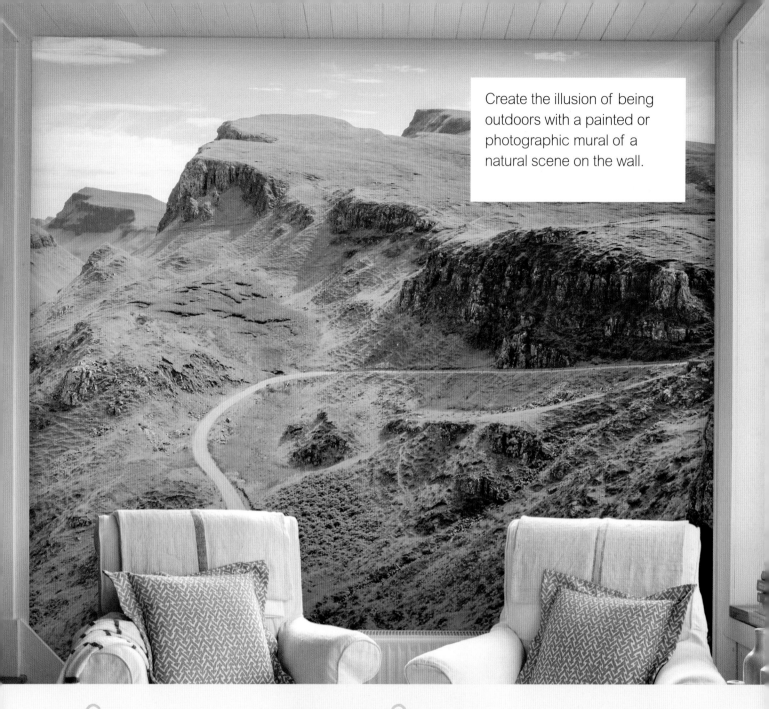

Create the illusion of being outdoors with a painted or photographic mural of a natural scene on the wall.

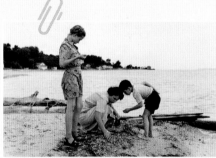

Beach bounty
Collect items that remind you of a favorite nature experience, perhaps from a vacation.

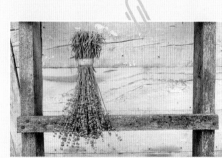

Dry some flowers
Trim the stems to the same length, tie with string, and hang out of direct sunlight.

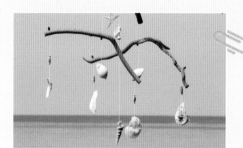

Make something
Use found natural objects to create something for the home, such as this mobile.

Make things with leaves

Leaves are abundant natural materials: use them to make simple items as a pleasant reminder of a country walk or as a celebration of your efforts in the garden.

How to do it

Take a large bag or bucket and gloves when you gather leaves; you may also need pruning shears or scissors.

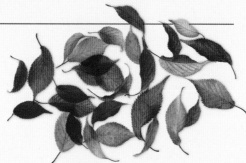

▲ Autumn leaves have wonderful colors but are more brittle, so handle them gently.

■ If using pressed leaves, collect them four weeks beforehand (see pages 158–159 for how to do this).

■ If you prefer to use fresh leaves, flatten them beneath a book overnight.

▶ There are lots of ways to use leaves. You may wish to collaborate on a project if you need assistance with the tricky parts.

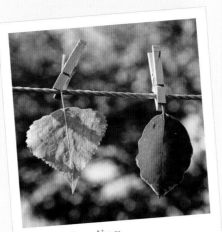

Create bunting

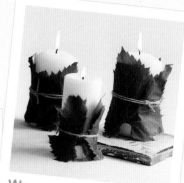

Wrap candles

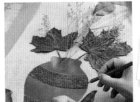

Make a card

AT A GLANCE

✓ Gentle activity

✓ 1 person

✓ Productivity/leisure

✓ Variable timeframe

✓ Moderate difficulty

! May include use of cutting tools or candles

! Beware of prickly plants when collecting leaves

HOW IT HELPS

A leaf project may give you the impetus to go on a nature walk or do some gardening, which brings its own benefits.

• Finding and choosing suitable leaves to use in a leaf project involves planning, organization, and decision-making.

• Completing craft projects require concentration, good hand-eye coordination, and fine motor skills.

• Using seasonal material such as leaves can help orientate you to time and the seasons.

TALK ABOUT...

Have you ever planted a tree yourself?

•

In which country are bonsai trees cultivated?

•

What other things could you make with leaves?

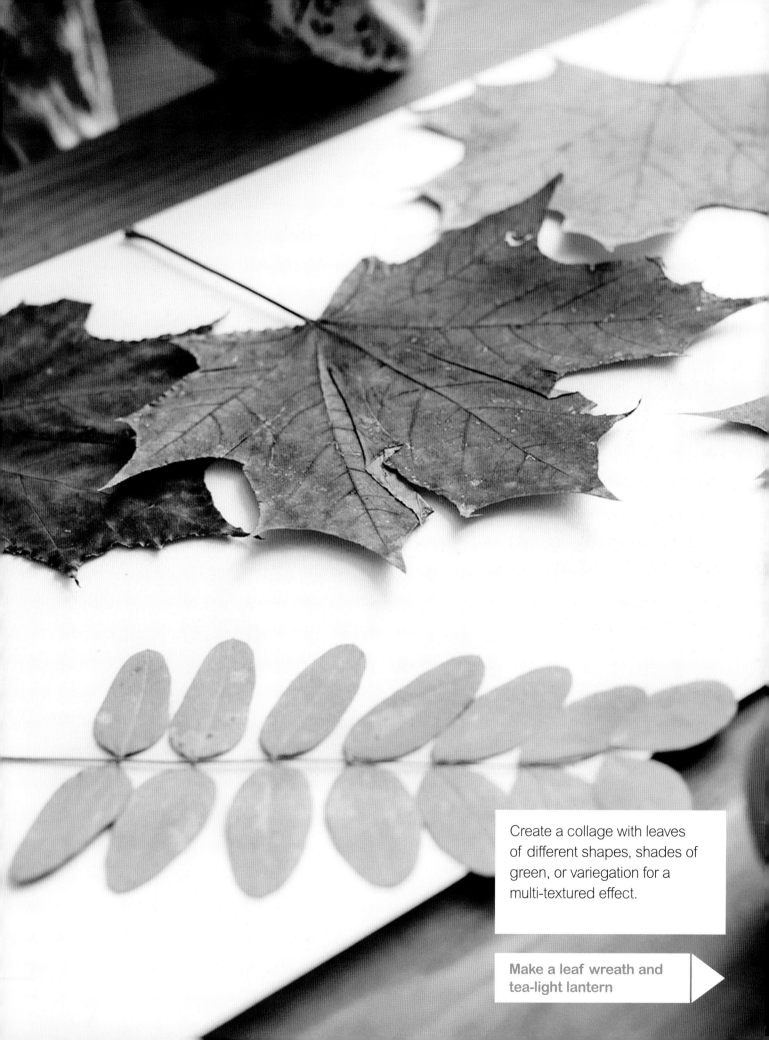

Create a collage with leaves of different shapes, shades of green, or variegation for a multi-textured effect.

Make a leaf wreath and tea-light lantern

Make a leaf wreath

Large, flat leaves are easier to handle and will make a bigger wreath. Once you have collected the leaves, trim off any stems with shears or scissors. Concentration is needed to thread leaves onto the wire, but this project can easily be put down and picked up again, if you feel the need to take a break.

WHAT YOU NEED
- 50–70 large leaves, freshly collected
- Pruning shears or scissors
- Garden wire, about 18 in (45 cm)
- Wire cutters

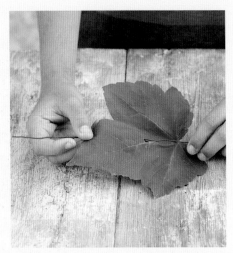 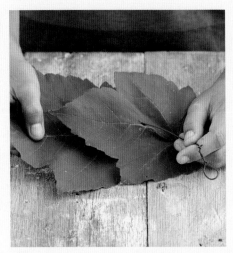 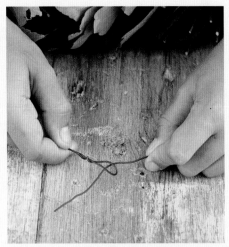

1 Fold the wire at one end and twist the end tightly to make a loop. Carefully push the other end of the wire through the center of a leaf.

2 Continue stringing leaves onto the wire. Make sure the stems all point inward. Push the leaves toward the bottom loop until you have used them all.

3 Push the sharp end of the wire through the loop. Pull the leaves into a circle. Fold the wire over the loop and twist to secure it. Trim off the excess wire.

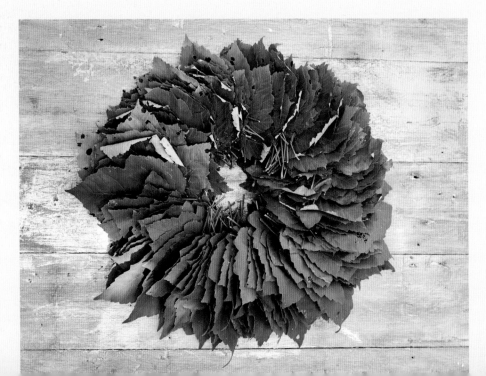

◄ Make a loop from the remainder of the wire length and use it to hang up your leaf wreath. The size of the wreath will depend upon the size of the leaves.

Make a tea-light lantern

Decorate jars with leaves and colorful ribbons to make these lanterns. You could use them as lovely table decorations or give them as gifts. If you use scented tea lights, they may evoke powerful memories. Evergreen leaves, such as ivy, can be collected at any time of year, or you could also use different leaves to reflect seasonal changes. Don't leave lanterns unattended when they are lit.

WHAT YOU NEED
- Several jam jars
- Strong wire and wire cutters
- Selection of leaves and seed heads, fresh or dried
- All-purpose glue
- Brush
- Scraps of ribbon
- Several tea lights

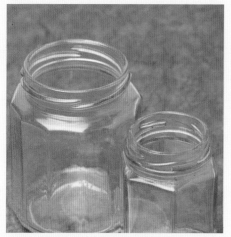

1 For each jar, cut a first piece of wire that is a little longer than the diameter of the jar neck.

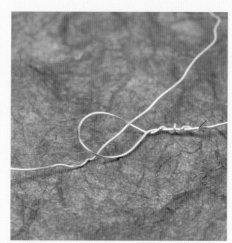

2 Cut a second piece of wire about 12 in (30 cm) long. Make a loop at either end. Thread the first piece through both loops.

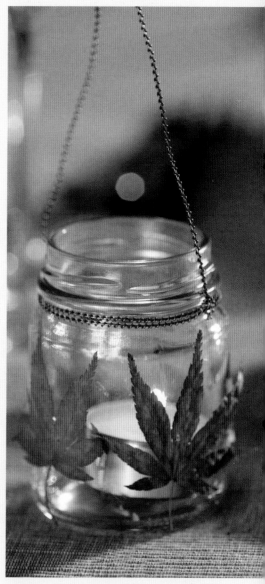

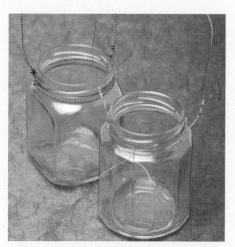

3 Wrap the short piece of wire around the jar neck. Wind the ends together. Position the loops so that the wire handle is upright.

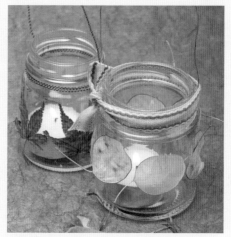

4 Glue leaves or seed heads onto the sides of the jar. Tie a ribbon around the neck. Put a tea light in the jar.

▲ Use leaves with bold, graphic shapes and bright colors for the greatest impact.

Sew something useful

Sewing can be both relaxing and productive, and if you've done it before, you may easily remember how to do it. Choose a project or task that is not too challenging so you can enjoy it.

If you have sewing experience, continue using your skills by making everything from decorative items to clothes, but you may choose to follow simpler patterns or designs.

■ Use fabrics that are easy to handle and avoid ones that are flimsy, shiny, or difficult to sew.

■ Try a plastic grid embroidery canvas: it is rigid, easy to hold and cut to shape, with holes big enough to take a thicker needle (easier to thread).

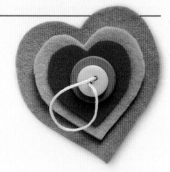

▲ Felt is an easy fabric to work with for small craft projects.

HOW IT HELPS

Sewing can quiet worrying thoughts and reduce anxiety. Completing a needlework project promotes confidence and self-esteem and gives you a sense of achievement.

• Sewing involves a range of physical skills, such as fine finger movement and good hand-eye coordination.

• This skill requires concentration, attention, decision-making, problem-solving, initiation, and the ability to follow sequences.

Embroidery
You may find cross stitch, embroidery, or needlepoint easier with thick thread and larger holes.

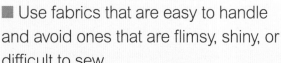

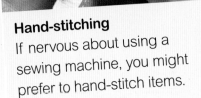

Hand-stitching
If nervous about using a sewing machine, you might prefer to hand-stitch items.

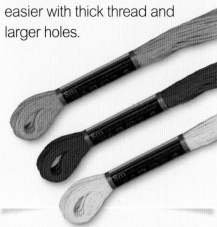

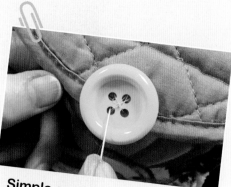

Simple sewing
Enjoy smaller sewing jobs, such as sewing on buttons, darning holes, and hemming.

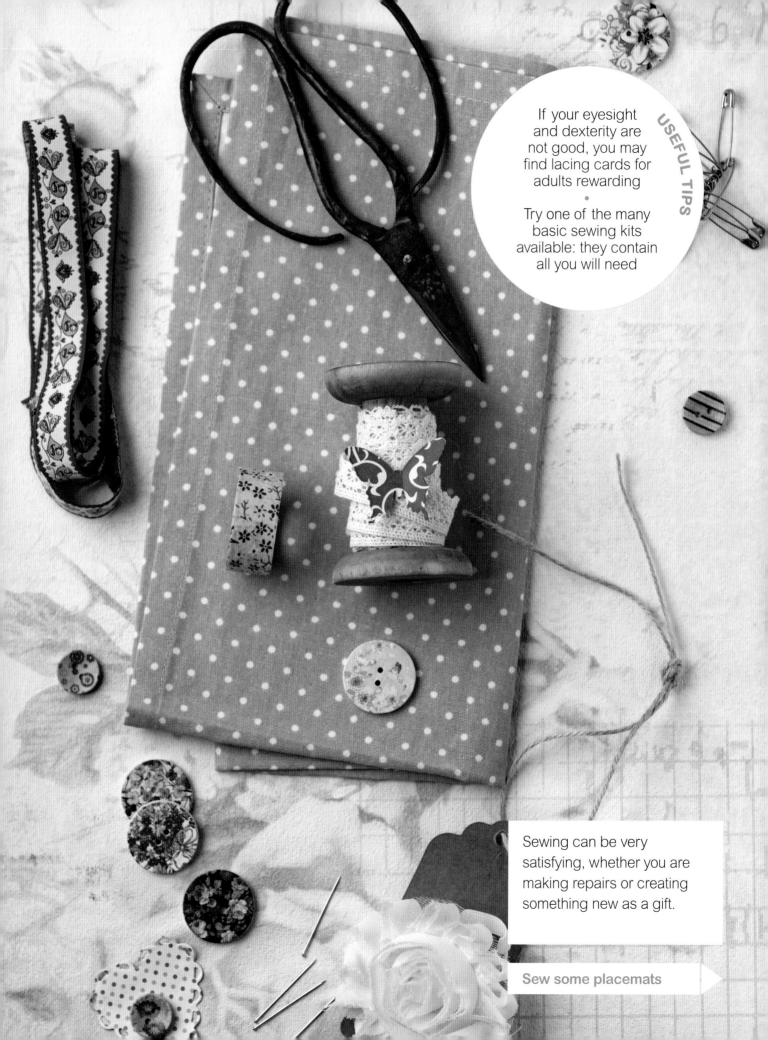

USEFUL TIPS

If your eyesight and dexterity are not good, you may find lacing cards for adults rewarding

Try one of the many basic sewing kits available: they contain all you will need

Sewing can be very satisfying, whether you are making repairs or creating something new as a gift.

Sew some placemats ▶

Choosing placemat colors and fabrics

If your visual perception is not what it was, placemats can help you to see the edges of your plate clearly, especially if the tabletop or tablecloth is a similar color to the plates. Look for plain, dark fabrics in colors that contrast with your dishes.

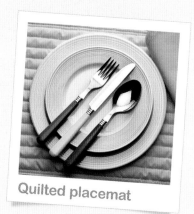

Quilted placemat

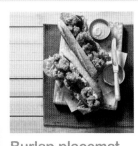

Burlap placemat

Sew some placemats

Making placemats is a great way to recycle old fabrics or even dish towels and tablecloths. The fabrics used here are red gingham and plain linen, but you could use any two colors of fabric. Cotton or linen is easiest to sew and to wash.

WHAT YOU NEED

- Interfacing
- 4 linen dish towels, or large piece of fabric, minimum 60 x 40in (153 x 102cm)
- Old gingham tablecloth, or large piece of fabric, minimum 60 x 40in (153 x 102cm)
- Tape measure
- Tailor's chalk or pencil
- Scissors
- Pins
- Needle
- Cotton thread
- Sewing machine equipped with spools of cotton thread (optional)

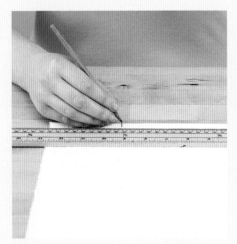

1 Measure and cut 4 pieces of interfacing, 4 pieces of linen, and 4 pieces of gingham. Each piece should be the same size: 13 x 9in (33 x 23cm).

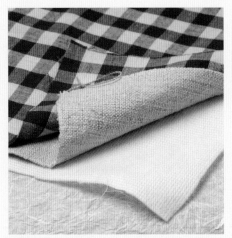

2 To make the first placemat, take a piece each of gingham and linen, with correct sides facing each other. Put them on a piece of interfacing.

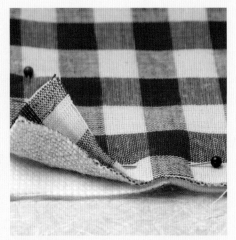

3 Make sure all the edges of the 3 pieces are aligned and pin them together. If you want, you can tack the edges for extra accuracy.

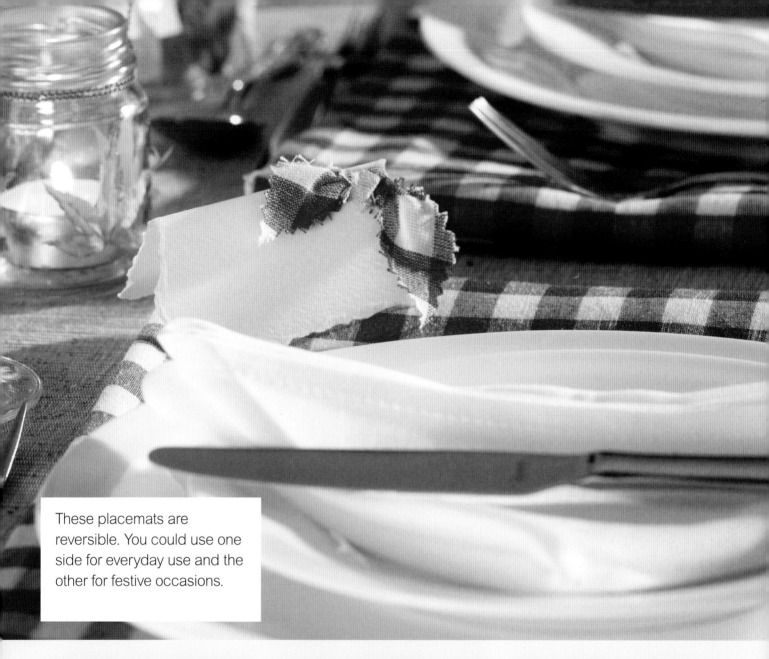

These placemats are reversible. You could use one side for everyday use and the other for festive occasions.

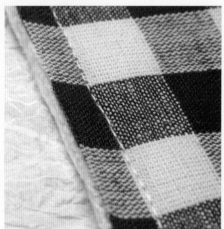

4 Sew a seam ½in (1 cm) wide along the edges, to join the fabrics together. Sew along 3 sides and half of the fourth side to leave a gap.

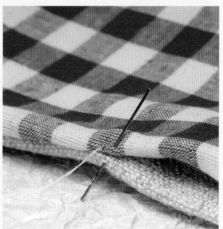

5 Turn the placemat inside out through the gap, so that the interfacing is hidden inside. Sew together the open edges to close the opening.

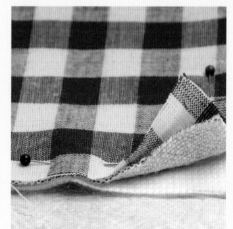

6 Use the remaining fabric pieces and repeat steps 2 to 5 in order to make another 3 placemats. You will then have made a set of 4 placemats.

Pick up the knitting needles

If you enjoy knitting or have knitted before, you may already realize its benefits. You can continue to enjoy this pastime with some simple adaptations.

How to do it

Don't struggle to follow complex patterns. If a pattern is too difficult, choose a simpler one. You may need someone to start you off by casting on for you.

■ You could enlarge the pattern on a photocopier to make it easier to read. Consider checking off each step as you complete it.

■ Larger needles are easier to hold and can be more comfortable to use.

▶ Look through old patterns and craft books for inspiration. You could make simple squares to create a patchwork blanket, or some baby clothes.

HOW IT HELPS

This craft uses a range of cognitive skills, including concentrating, understanding and following instructions, initiating and sequencing, and problem-solving.

• Knitting uses procedural memory if you have knitted previously.

• It is rhythmic and repetitious, and therefore can be relaxing.

• Knitting requires good hand-eye coordination and dexterity.

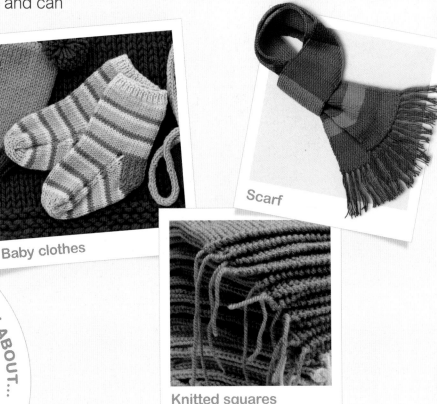

Baby clothes

Scarf

Knitted squares

TALK ABOUT...

Did you help to wind balls of yarn from skeins?

What was the first thing you knitted or crocheted?

Think of some knitting stitches and techniques

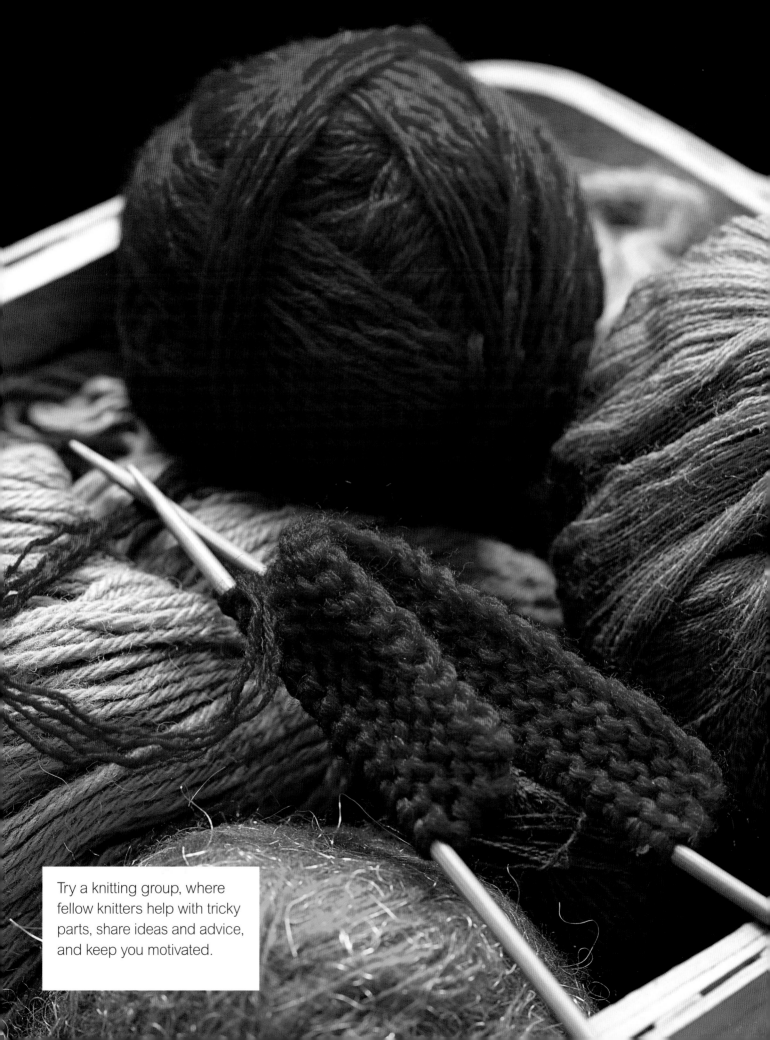

Try a knitting group, where fellow knitters help with tricky parts, share ideas and advice, and keep you motivated.

Make a fidget cuff

A fidget cuff is a rewarding item to make, since you can use it yourself or make a few to donate to a hospital or dementia charity. They are relatively simple to produce.

How to do it

Gather everything you need before you start, including any odd balls of yarn and bits of bric-a-brac.

■ You might prefer to share the tasks involved with someone else. You can also do a little bit at a time.

■ Adapt the design of the cuff to your strengths and abilities, for example, you could disguise the odd dropped stitch with embellishments.

▶ Search through your sewing basket and button box for any items with interesting textures, colors, and shapes.

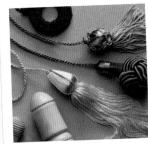
Tassels

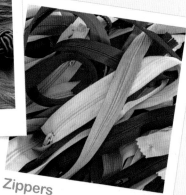
Zippers

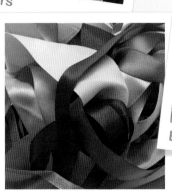
Ribbons

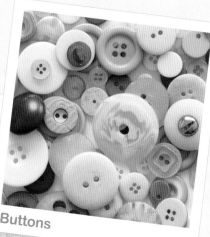
Buttons

TALK ABOUT...

What other items could you use to decorate a fidget cuff?

Think of fragrant items you could slip into a pocket on the fidget cuff

What crackly item could you add to the cuff to stimulate hearing?

AT A GLANCE

✓ Gentle activity

✓ 1 or more people

✓ Productivity

✓ 3–4 hours

✓ Moderate difficulty

HOW IT HELPS

Doing something practical and useful to support others can give you a great sense of achievement and pride.

• If you have always knitted, you use procedural memory to complete this activity.

• You are free to create your own design, so you can enjoy the process without any anxiety about doing it incorrectly.

• Creating the cuff involves cognitive skills following a sequence, concentrating, and making choices and decisions.

• Colorful fidget cuffs stimulate vision and the tactile decorations stimulate the sense of touch. They can also alleviate agitation.

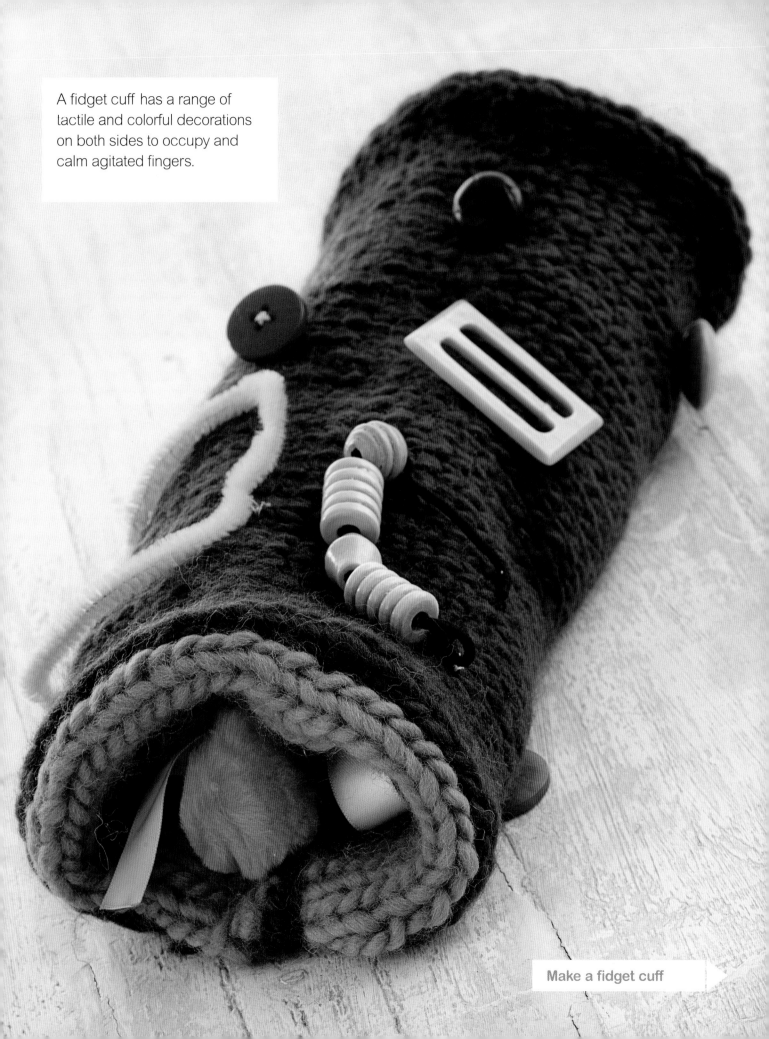

A fidget cuff has a range of tactile and colorful decorations on both sides to occupy and calm agitated fingers.

Make a fidget cuff ▶

Collect your decorations

You will need 14 to 18 tactile items to decorate the cuff. These could be: felt items, buttons, fabric loops, hair scrunchies, pom-poms, ribbons, tassels, and plastic curtain rings threaded onto a rope. Don't use anything with sharp points or edges or that is too small to grasp easily. Things that open and close, such as zippers or velcro, add a touch element.

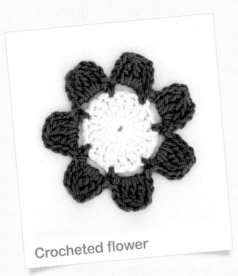

Crocheted flower

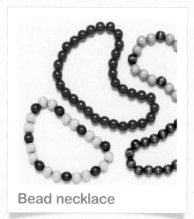

Bead necklace

Make a fidget cuff

This cuff is made from a double layer of knitting, with two colors of yarn so the inside and outside are different colors. However, you could use just one color of yarn if you prefer. It is the smallest size you could make, but you could make a roomier one by adding rows in both colors.

WHAT YOU NEED
- 2 x 150g balls of thick yarn
- 1 pair large knitting needles, size 7–9
- Tapestry needle
- Scissors
- Sewing needle
- Button thread
- 14–18 tactile items

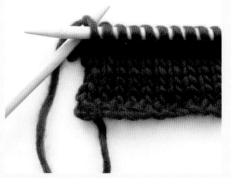

1 Cast on 48 stitches—garter or stocking stitch is easiest—or enough to start knitting a piece about 12 in (30 cm) wide.

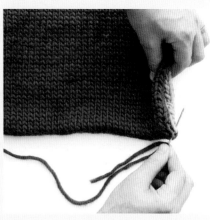

5 Use a tapestry needle and yarn to sew together the edges of one side of the folded square.

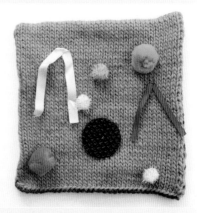

9 Sew the remaining, softer items to the other side of the knitted square (this will be the inside).

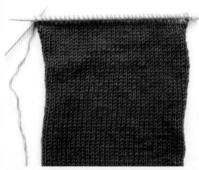

2 When the piece is 12 in (30 cm) long, switch to the second color of yarn, by knotting the new yarn to the old.

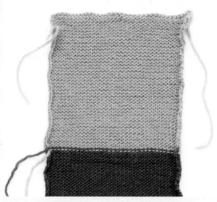

3 Continue knitting until the piece is 24 in (60 cm) long. Then cast off, or get someone to help you to cast off.

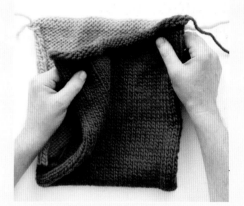

4 Fold the piece of knitting in half lengthwise with the pearl side facing inward to make a double-thickness square.

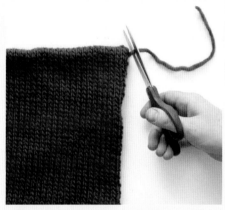

6 Sew together the other two open sides of the square. At the end, knot the yarn and cut neatly.

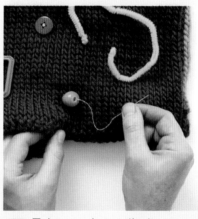

7 Take each tactile item and sew it securely to one side of the knitted square. Cut off any loose ends of thread.

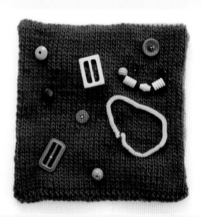

8 Sew 7–9 of the most bulky tactile items to one side of the knitted square (this will be the outside).

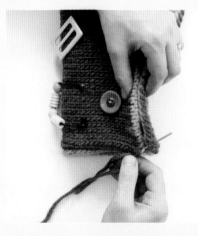

10 Sew the two opposite sides of the square, with a tapestry needle, to form a tube.

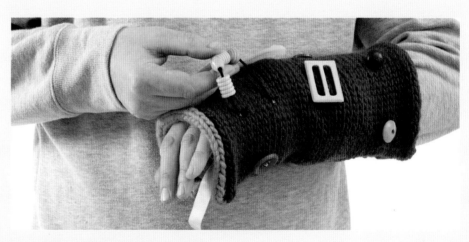

11 The finished fidget cuff has tactile decorations on both the outside and inside.

Make a sensory blanket

Sensory blankets are decorated with a variety of objects to stimulate vision, touch, and even smell. Make one for a friend or for yourself.

How to do it

There is no "correct" way to make a sensory blanket—each is unique. The items you use as decorations will depend on your taste and what is available.

■ People who have Alzheimer's disease have diminished sensitivity to visual contrast, so consider a bright color of fleece.

▲ You could adapt this idea to make a sensory cushion or apron.

■ Make your fleece at least 40 x 32 inches (100 x 80 cm) or big enough to cover the lap.

■ Once you have chosen suitable items, space them all out on the blanket, in the area that would be over your lap.

■ Sew each item securely in place. Dental floss is great for sewing on buttons.

▶ Choose a washable blanket in a bright color, but avoid busy patterns. Use a close-knit texture and medium weight, such as fleece.

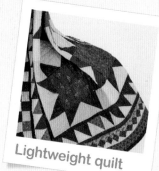
Lightweight quilt

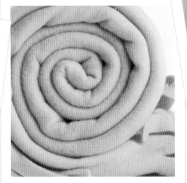
Synthetic fleece

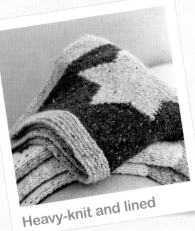
Heavy-knit and lined

HOW IT HELPS

The blanket can provide sensory comfort, which will result in emotional comfort.

• Assembling items, designing, and making a sensory blanket involves cognitive skills such as making choices, planning, organizing, and concentration.

• Sewing the items to the blanket is good practice for your manual dexterity, fine motor skills, and hand-eye coordination.

• This creative activity and its completion brings a sense of achievement.

• Stroking and fiddling with the attachments on the blanket keeps restless hands busy, is soothing, and reduces agitation.

Choose some sensory items

Embellish the blanket with "doing things" such as a button flap, zippers, and velcro to open and close. Add things to stroke, twirl, pull at, or put things in. Try to include different textures, such as fluffy, hard, or velvety, as well as fragrant items, for example a bouquet garni sachet.

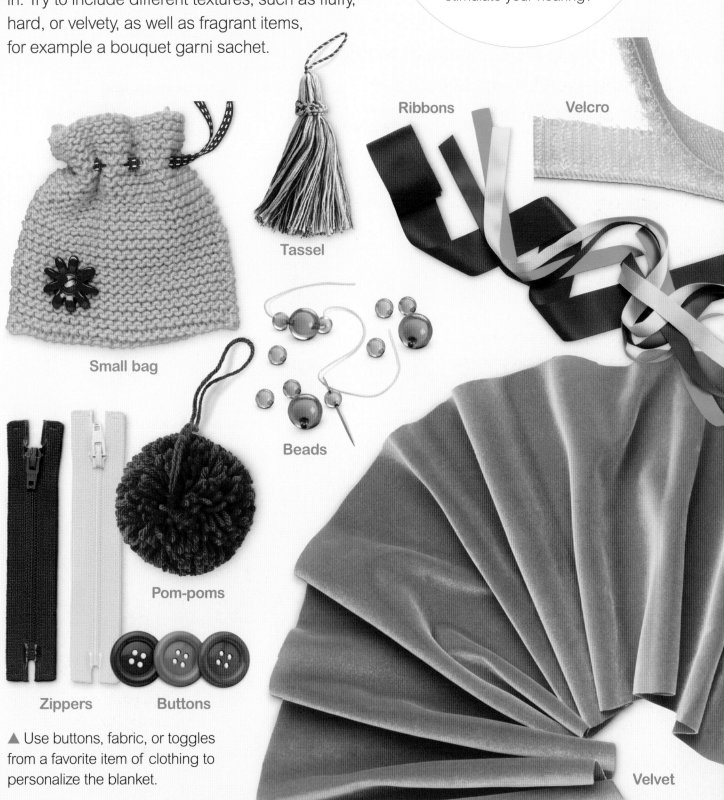

TALK ABOUT…

What else could you use to personalize a blanket?

Do you have a favorite texture?

What can you add to the blanket that would stimulate your hearing?

Tassel

Ribbons

Velcro

Small bag

Beads

Zippers

Pom-poms

Buttons

Velvet

▲ Use buttons, fabric, or toggles from a favorite item of clothing to personalize the blanket.

Make festive decorations

Make your own decorations to celebrate a special occasion such as a birthday, homecoming, garden party, annual festival, or anniversary.

How to do it

Think about your theme and color scheme: for example primary colors for a child's birthday, pale greens and yellows for spring, or silver for a wedding.

■ Banners are easy to make and great for outdoor festivities. Put up tea-light lanterns (see page 187) for use in the evening.

■ You may want to share this project. Each person could take responsibility for a particular part.

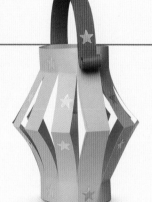

▲ Paper lanterns are easy to make. You can decorate them to make them more colorful.

AT A GLANCE

✓ Sedentary

✓ 1 or more people

✓ Productivity/leisure

✓ Variable timeframe

✓ Variable difficulty

! May involve use of scissors or stapler

HOW IT HELPS

Making decorations can be easy, and allows you to be creative without the pressure of making something that has to last.

• You use a range of physical and mental skills to complete this type of project, including decision-making, concentrating, planning, organizing, following sequences, and paying attention.

• Completing the decorations will give you a sense of achievement and increase your self-esteem.

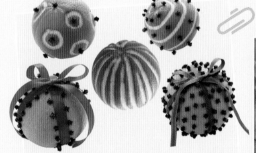

Orange pomander
Make fragrant pomanders from dried oranges that are studded with cloves.

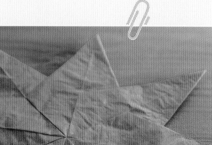

Paper stars
Search books or online to find detailed instructions on how to make other fun paper decorations, like these stars.

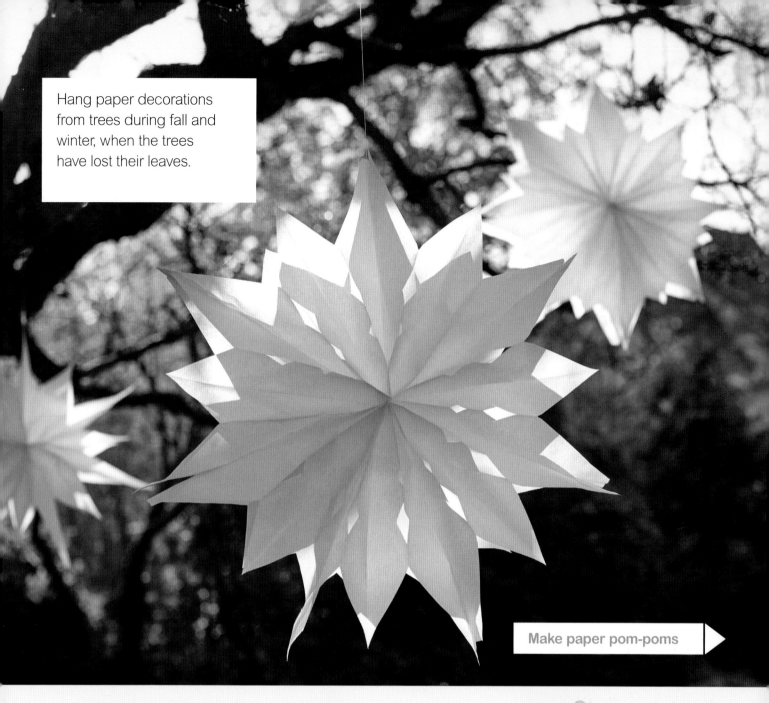

Hang paper decorations from trees during fall and winter, when the trees have lost their leaves.

Make paper pom-poms ➡

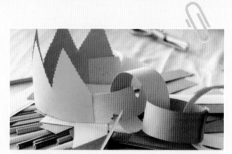

Paper chains
Take paper strips, about 8 x ½ in (20 cm x 1.2 cm) wide. Glue or staple to join the loops.

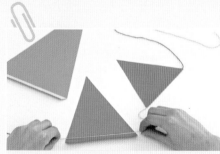

Banners
Cut out triangles of colored paper or cloth, and glue or sew them to a piece of string.

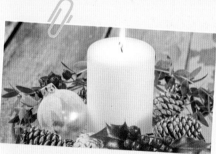

Pine centerpiece
For a table decoration, put a candle in a circular glass dish and add some pine sprigs, baubles, and cones.

Make paper pom-poms

Each sheet makes one hand-sized pom-pom. Make the pom-poms in your theme color or in different hues, and hang them up as a bunting or on trees. You could also hang up a group of them above the center of a table.

WHAT YOU NEED
- Sheets of colored tissue paper, each 30 x 20 in (75 x 50 cm)
- Scissors
- Metal spoon
- 20 in (50 cm) pieces of florists' wire
- Invisible thread

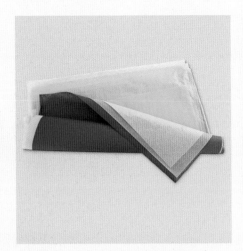

1 Take 1 or more sheets and fold them neatly in half. Fold them in half width-ways twice more. Unfold the sheets.

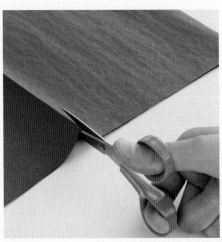

2 Cut each sheet along the fold marks to divide the sheet into 8 smaller sheets. Stack the 8 sheets on top of each other.

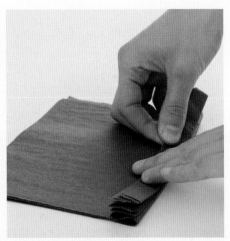

3 Start at a short end. Fold the tissue stack into ½ in (1.2 cm) wide accordion folds. Crease folds by pressing with a spoon.

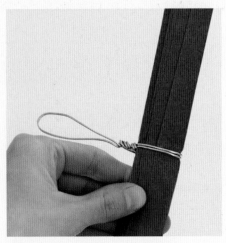

5 Open the looped end of the wire. Tuck in the wire ends so that they don't stick out.

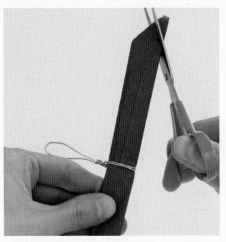

6 Cut 2 corners of one end of the paper strip to make it pointed. Cut the other end in the same way.

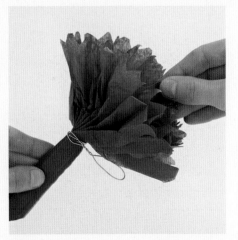

7 Gently pull the outermost fold of paper from one end of the strip. Pull out each layer of paper until you reach the center.

Make giant pom-poms

For really impressive decorations, use eight whole sheets of tissue paper for each pom-pom. Put the sheets flat on top of each other. Then follow steps 1 to 8, but when you get to step 3, make the folds bigger—about 1 in (2.5 cm) wide.

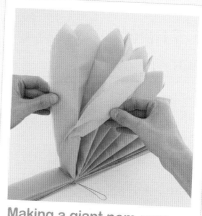

Making a giant pom-pom

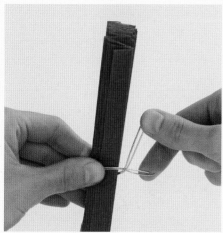

4 Bend a piece of florist's wire in half. Bend it again and twist it firmly around the center of the folded paper.

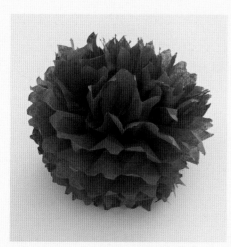

8 Pull out all the layers of paper on the other end of the strip until you have a pom-pom shape.

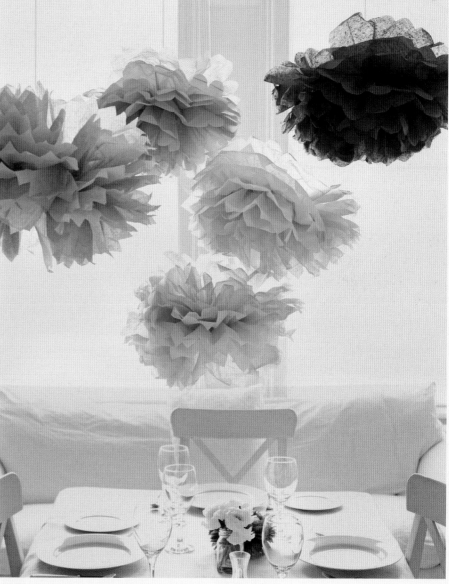

▲ Tie a piece of invisible thread to each wire loop and hang up the pom-poms. Group several pom-poms at different heights to make the decorations look more striking.

Make memory labels and signs

Creating your own customized labels and directional signs can compensate for memory problems and help you to remain independent for as long as possible.

How to do it

First, identify the things or basic routines that you are finding frustrating to locate or remember. It can help to talk this through with a family member.

■ Think of where each label and sign can be placed so that it is visible but does not interfere with opening and closing doors or drawers.

■ Labels with simple instructions on how to use appliances, such as the washing machine, will help you to use them safely for longer.

■ Do not make too many signs as you will stop paying attention to them.

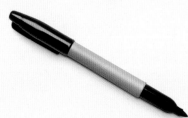

▲ Use a thick, black marker to color in an arrow or to write key words or basic steps to a routine in bold print.

AT A GLANCE

✓ Gentle activity

✓ 1 person

✓ Self care/productivity

✓ Variable timeframe

✓ Easy

! May involve use of scissors

HOW IT HELPS

Creating memory labels and signs can make you feel empowered, because they help you to remain independent.

• Signs help to orientate you in and around the home, with visual prompts of what is behind each closed door.

• Some frustrations caused by memory problems are alleviated, which is good for confidence and well-being.

• Visual reminders can prompt long-term procedural memories and help with initiating tasks.

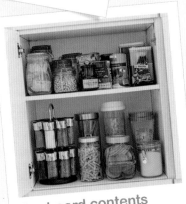

Kitchen

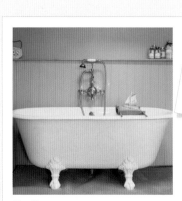

Bathroom

Cupboard contents

▲ You could use memory labels and signs around the home to remind you of where rooms or things are, or of basic instructions.

TALK ABOUT...

What signs would you like to make?

•

Consider if a pocket-sized reminder card might be useful, for example one with your address or a contact telephone number to take when away from home

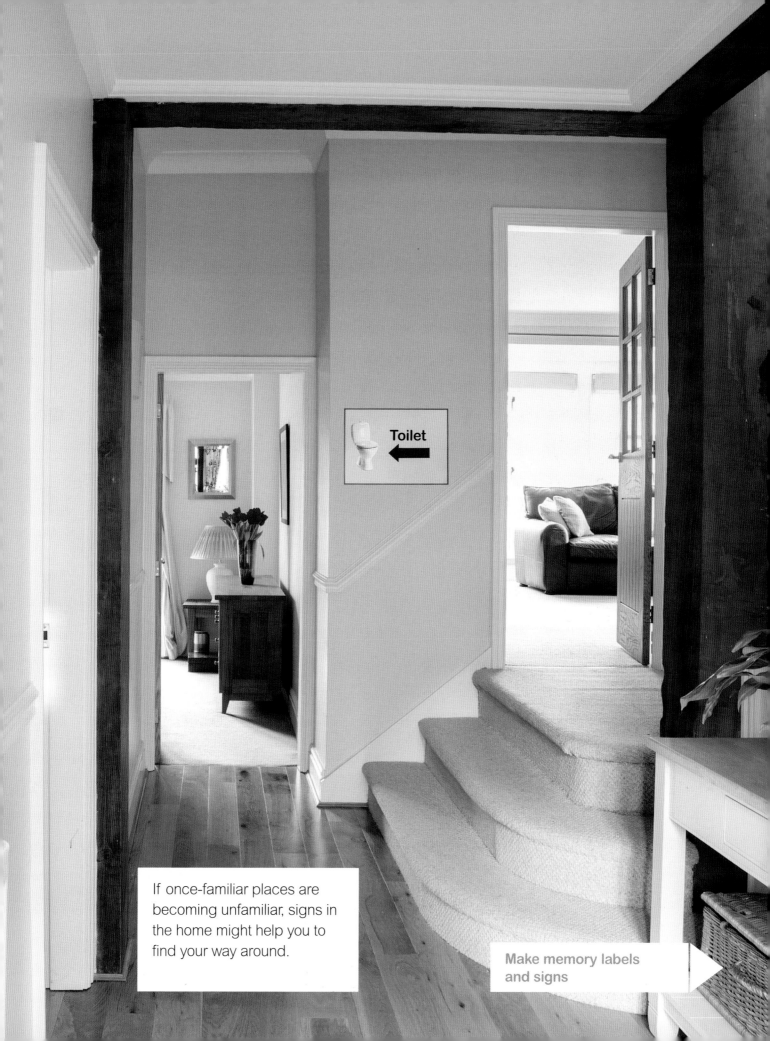

Toilet

If once-familiar places are becoming unfamiliar, signs in the home might help you to find your way around.

Make memory labels and signs

Make a list

Before you make any labels or signs, list all the items, rooms, or instructions you think you may need to be reminded of. Think about labeling cupboard doors and drawers to remind you what's inside them. Also make labels to remind you of the essentials you need every time you leave the house.

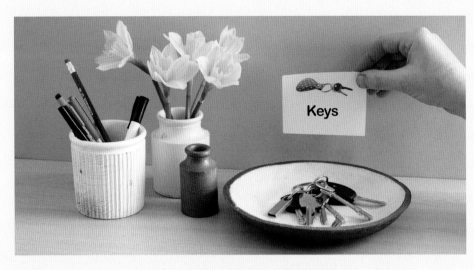

▲ If you're misplacing your keys often, make a sign to remind you to always store them in the same place.

Make memory labels

Each memory label has to stand out against the surface you will be sticking it on. Use brightly colored cards or labels for pale surfaces and white ones for dark surfaces. If you're making instructions, think about where the cards will be placed once made.

WHAT YOU NEED
- Printed images or magazines
- Scissors
- White or colored cards or large sticky labels
- Glue stick
- Thick, black marker
- Laminator (optional)
- Adhesive putty

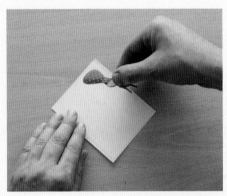

1 Find an image to represent the object you want to label. Cut out the image and glue it to the card or sticky label.

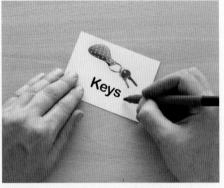

2 Use a thick, black marker to write the name of the objects you want to remember on the label.

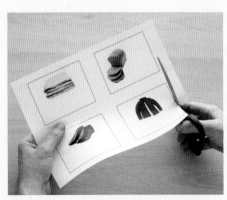

3 You may prefer to design your labels on a computer and print them out. Cut out each label and stick them on a card.

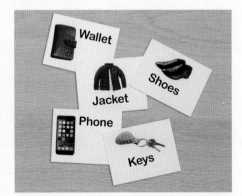

4 When you've finished all the labels, laminate them to keep them clean, or use putty or tape to stick them in place.

Make memory signs

Make signs with an arrow to go on the wall or ones without arrows for doors. You could also photograph familiar items from each room to print out on paper. You may need help with this. Laminate signs to keep them clean.

WHAT YOU NEED

- Magazines
- Camera or smartphone
- Computer with printer
- Scissors
- Pieces of colored card stock (yellow is good)
- Thick, black marker
- Glue stick
- Laminator (optional)
- Adhesive putty

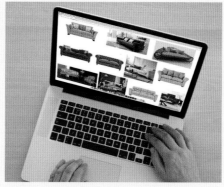

1 Look in magazines or online for images to represent a key, recognizable feature of each room in your home.

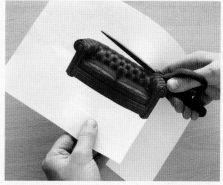

2 For example, a sofa could represent your living room or an oven for your kitchen. Print and cut out the images.

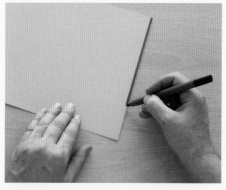

3 Outline each card in thick, black marker around all 4 edges. Turn the paper to a landscape orientation.

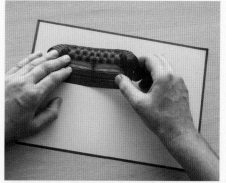

4 Glue each image on to one of the cards. Leave space below each image for text and an arrow (if needed).

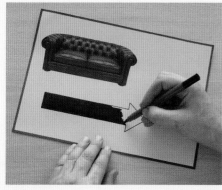

5 Add an arrow pointing in the right direction, and then write down the name of the room to which the sign will point.

6 When the signs are all done, use putty to stick each sign on a wall or door, at shoulder height where you can see it easily.

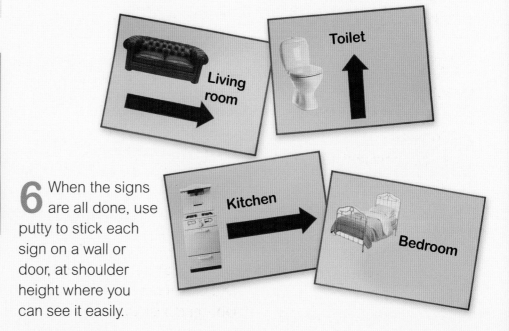

Keep cooking

Whether you find cooking, preparing, and serving food a chore or a pleasure, it is good to continue using your skills. It will help you to feel useful in everyday life.

How to do it

You may find that your tastes change, so now is the time to try new flavors. If things are getting more difficult for you, there are ways to simplify cooking.

■ Write down how to cook family favorites or find simple recipes from cookbooks or online.

■ Buy frozen, canned, or prepared ingredients. Or get ready-made meals instead of preparing fresh ingredients.

■ Concentrate on one thing at a time so that the task doesn't become overwhelming.

■ You might want to recreate dishes that remind you of past holidays or special occasions.

AT A GLANCE

✓ Active

✓ 1 or more people

✓ Self-care/productivity

✓ Variable timeframe

✓ Variable difficulty

! Variable safety

HOW IT HELPS

Being involved with preparing food will stimulate all your senses. Seeing, touching, smelling, and tasting food—even hearing food sizzling in a pan—can sharpen the appetite.

• You use cognitive skills such as concentrating, following sequences, and problem-solving to choose what to make, to plan, and to prepare meals.

• Recreating favorite recipes uses procedural memory.

• Celebrating special occasions with food can trigger your emotional memories.

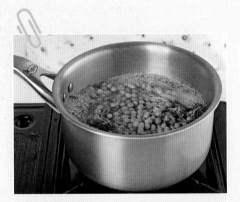

Hot food
Be aware of safety issues: take care while handling hot food if you have difficulties with vision or hand-eye coordination.

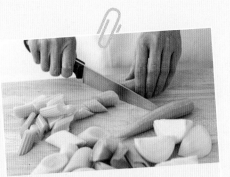

Share the workload
If you don't want to cook alone, help out with tasks such as peeling potatoes, beating eggs, or chopping vegetables.

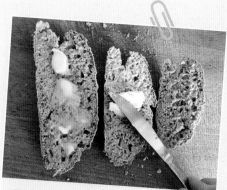

Easy tasks
Keep preparing simple snacks and drinks, such as making sandwiches and buttering bread, as long as you are able.

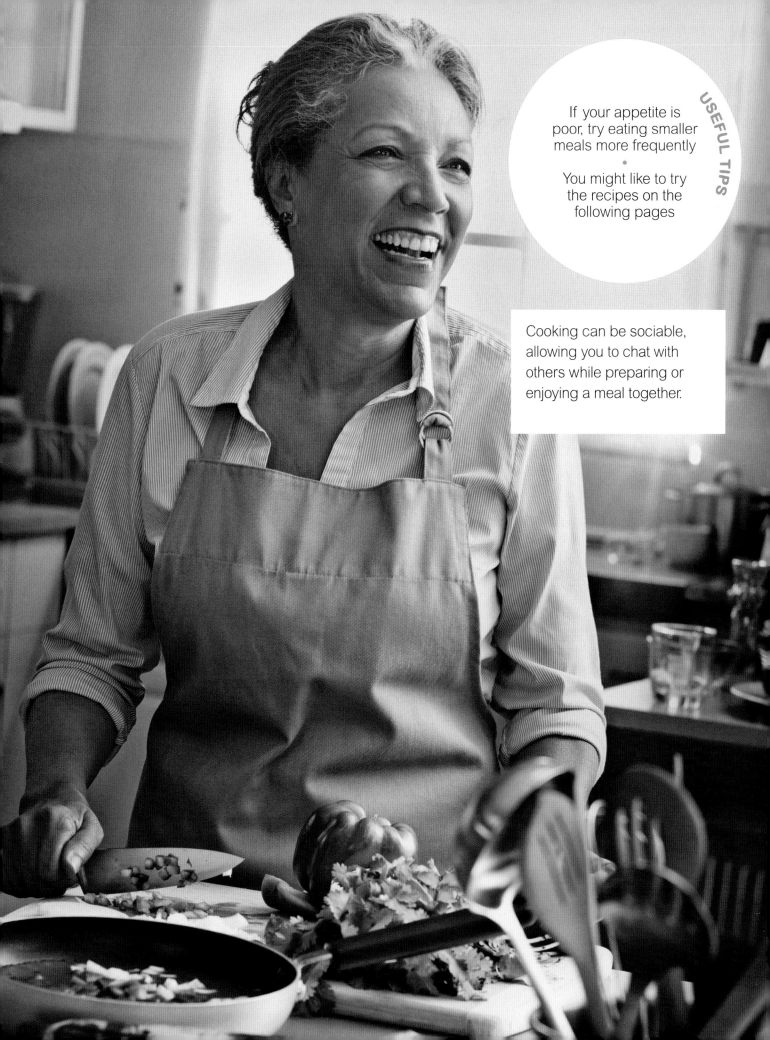

If your appetite is poor, try eating smaller meals more frequently

·

You might like to try the recipes on the following pages

Cooking can be sociable, allowing you to chat with others while preparing or enjoying a meal together.

Healthy salads

Preparing light snacks and meals helps to maintain your independence. Healthy salads can be quick and easy to make.

How to do it

Salads can be as simple or as elaborate as you want to make them, so choose a recipe to suit your ability.

■ Make a basic salad from a few salad leaves; add tomatoes, cucumber, and your favorite dressing.

■ Try adding grated raw vegetables, such as carrots, and sliced peppers and onions.

■ Adding ingredients to a premade salad is even easier.

▲ You could add some fish to your salad for a healthy meal.

▶ There are lots of salad recipes to try, or just make up your own from your favorite salad vegetables.

HOW IT HELPS

Making a salad helps you to maintain a balanced diet, which can benefit brain and overall health.

• Making even a basic salad exercises cognitive skills of planning, organizing, following sequences, concentrating, initiating, and completing tasks.

• Selecting favorite ingredients or experimenting with new flavors helps with decision-making and choice.

• Moving around in the kitchen keeps you mobile and supple. You use fine motor skills to peel, chop, and prepare salad.

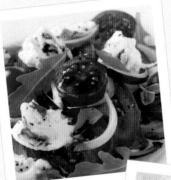
Tomato salad

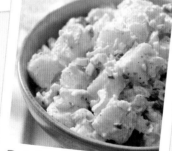
Potato salad

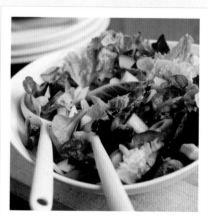
Green salad

TALK ABOUT...

What is your favorite salad dressing?

Do you love or hate salads?

Did you ever grow your own salad vegetables?

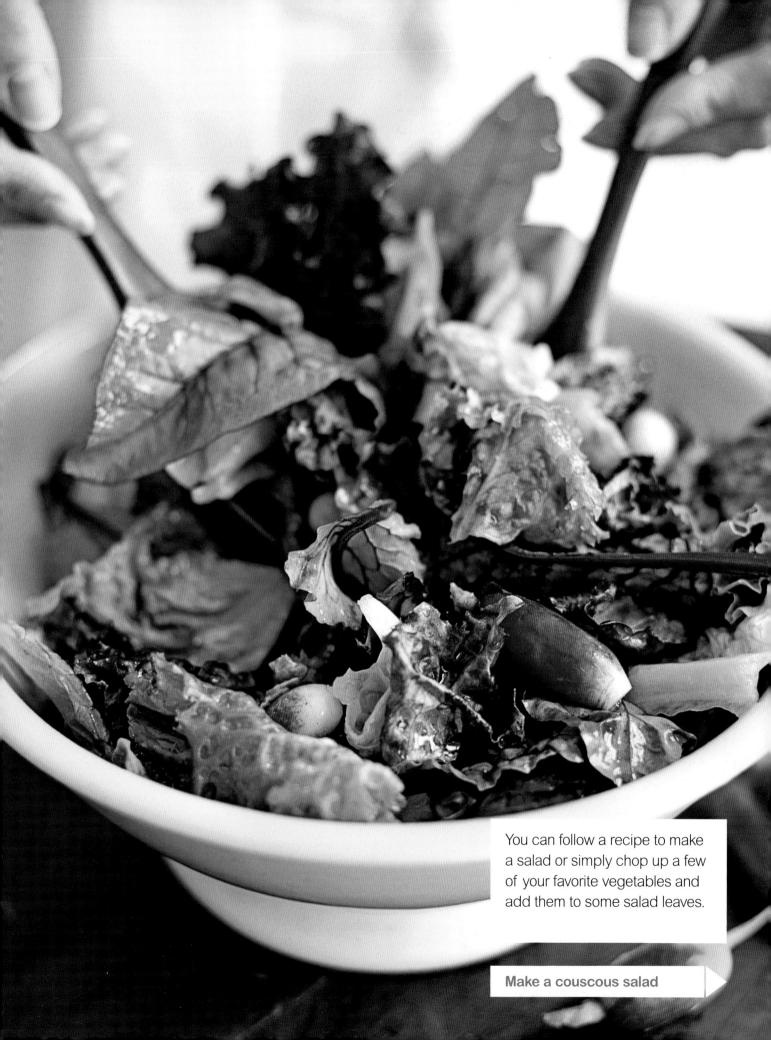

You can follow a recipe to make a salad or simply chop up a few of your favorite vegetables and add them to some salad leaves.

Make a couscous salad

Make a couscous salad

Salads like this one, with pasta, rice, couscous, or other grains, make a filling meal. If you don't like feta, try a different cheese. Why not try different flavors by adding your favorite salad ingredients to the basic couscous? The easiest way to prepare vegetable stock is to use bouillon cubes and add hot water: just follow the instructions on the package. This recipe serves four and takes 20 minutes to prepare.

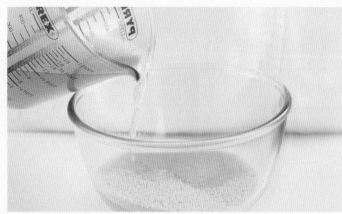

1 Prepare 1 cup (250 ml) of hot vegetable stock. Put the couscous in a large bowl and pour the hot stock over it.

WHAT YOU NEED

- 3 bowls
- Measuring cup
- Fork
- Chopping board
- Knife
- Teaspoon
- Wooden spoon
- Fine grater or lemon zester
- Lemon squeezer

RECIPE INGREDIENTS

- 1 cup (250 ml) hot vegetable stock
- ¾ cup (170 g) couscous
- 9 oz (250 g) cherry tomatoes
- Small red onion
- Half cucumber
- Medium-sized pomegranate (or 2 packets pre-peeled pomegranate seeds)
- 1 lemon
- 2 tbsp olive oil
- 7 oz (200 g) feta cheese, crumbled
- Large bunch fresh mint, chopped

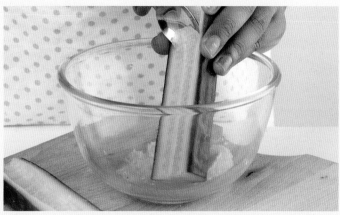

4 Cut the cucumber in half lengthwise. With a teaspoon, scoop out the seeds; discard them. Use a knife to dice the cucumber.

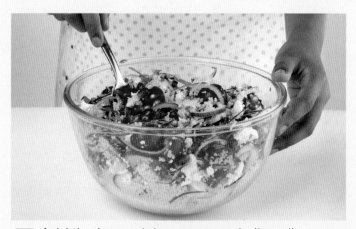

7 Add the lemon juice, zest, and olive oil to the couscous and stir. Then add all the other ingredients.

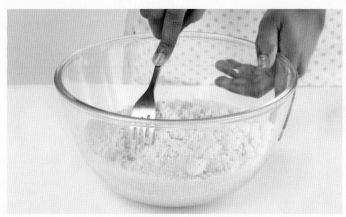

2 Stir the couscous well with the fork until the stock is absorbed (about 5 minutes). Put the couscous aside to cool.

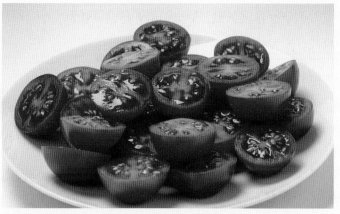

3 Wash and dry the cherry tomatoes and cut them all in half. Peel the onion, cut it in half, and then slice both halves of the onion thinly.

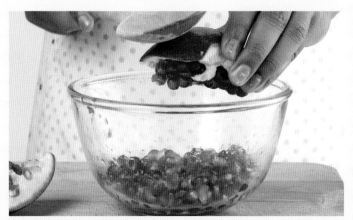

5 Cut the pomegranate in half. Hold each half over a bowl; tap with the wooden spoon so the seeds fall in the bowl.

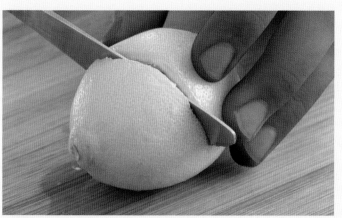

6 Grate the lemon rind or scrape it with a zester to make zest. Slice the lemon in half and squeeze each half to extract the juice.

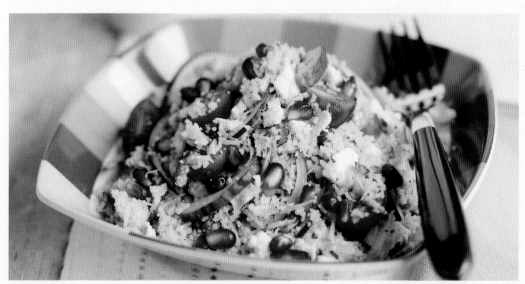

◀ Serve the salad right away. Alternatively, put in the fridge to eat later: label with the date and eat within two days.

Make sweet treats

Making sweet treats is a fun way to cook, although you'll want to limit your intake, since sweets aren't good for brain health.

How to do it

Before you start, set out all the ingredients and utensils you need.

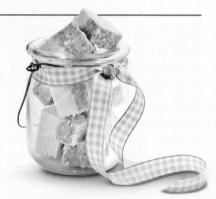

■ Prepare your work surface. You may prefer to sit at a table for the mixing stages, rather than stand at a counter.

■ Weigh all the ingredients and place them in separate bowls.

▲ Put some of your homemade treats in a jar, and tie it with ribbon to make a pretty gift.

■ You could make the treats with younger members of your family and pass on your cooking tips.

HOW IT HELPS

This project helps with dexterity as well as giving you a sense of achievement and boosting your confidence and self-esteem.

• Following a recipe requires cognitive skills, such as planning, calculating weights, and following sequences.

• If this is a familiar activity, it also uses procedural memory.

• Cooking stimulates touch and smell—the most powerful sense for creating emotional responses and triggering memories.

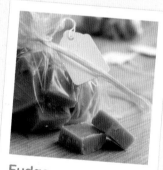

Fudge

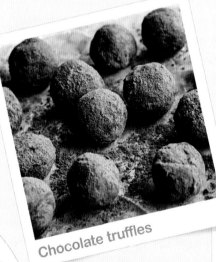

Chocolate truffles

◄ Whether you are a novice or you have always enjoyed baking, the best part of making sweets and cakes is tasting the results.

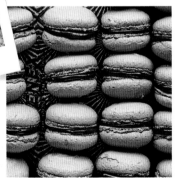

Macarons

TALK ABOUT...

What are your favorite sweets?

•

What sweet treats have you made before?

•

Do you prefer sweet or savory food?

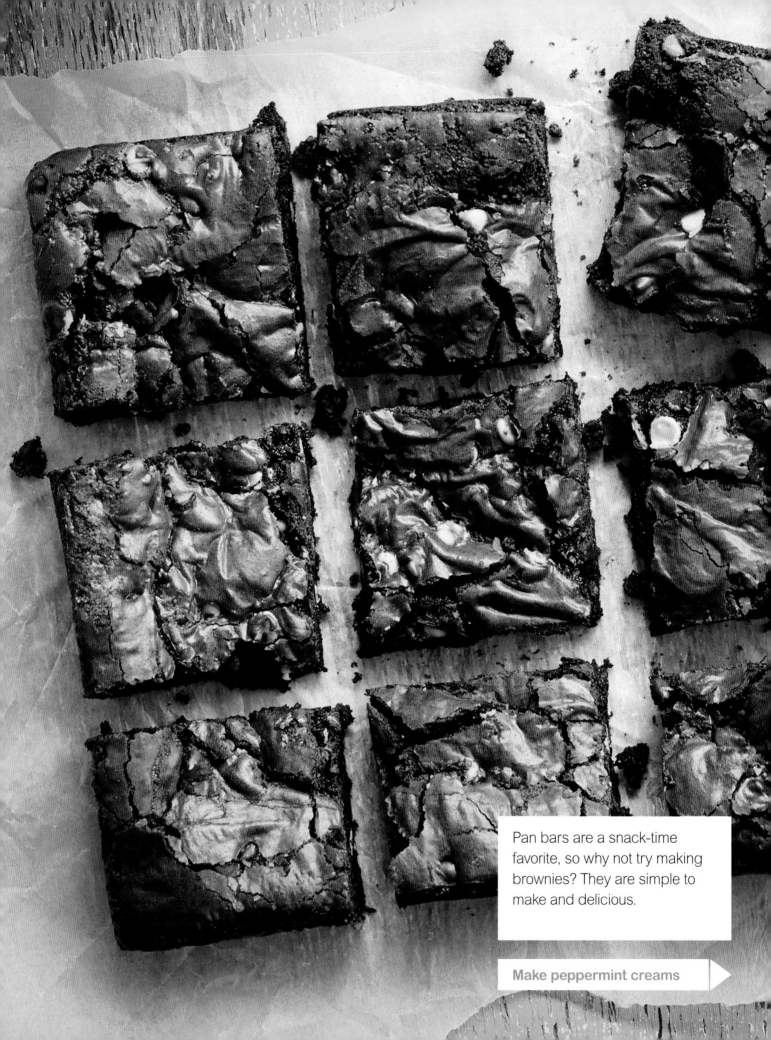

Pan bars are a snack-time favorite, so why not try making brownies? They are simple to make and delicious.

Make peppermint creams ⟶

Plain mint creams

If you want to avoid working with hot chocolate, as shown in this recipe, simply make these sweets as plain mints. You could also make different colors of mints by using a selection of food coloring.

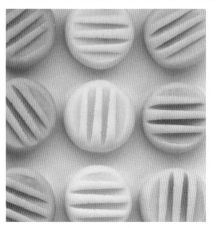

Plain mints

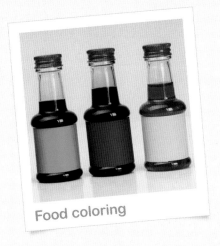

Food coloring

Make peppermint creams

This recipe is easy to follow and makes delicious sweets. It takes 20–30 minutes to make 60 peppermint creams, so there will be plenty to go around. Follow these instructions carefully.

WHAT YOU NEED
- Sieve
- Large mixing bowl
- Metal tablespoon
- Flat baking pan
- Parchment paper
- Rolling pin
- 2 in (5 cm) round cookie cutter
- Heatproof bowl
- Heatproof spatula
- Saucepan

RECIPE INGREDIENTS
- 1 lb (450 g) powdered sugar
- ½ cup (120 ml) sweetened condensed milk
- 3 drops peppermint oil
- 3 drops green food coloring
- 5½ oz (150 g) dark chocolate

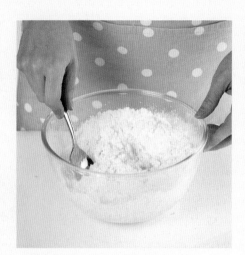

1 Sift the powdered sugar into the mixing bowl. Add the condensed milk. Stir with a metal spoon until the mixture is crumbly.

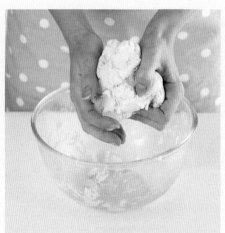

2 Add the peppermint oil and the food coloring—take care not to add too much. Knead the mix until it has a smooth, firm texture.

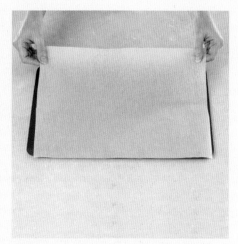

3 Line the baking tray with parchment paper. Dust your work surface by shaking a sieve with a little powdered sugar over it.

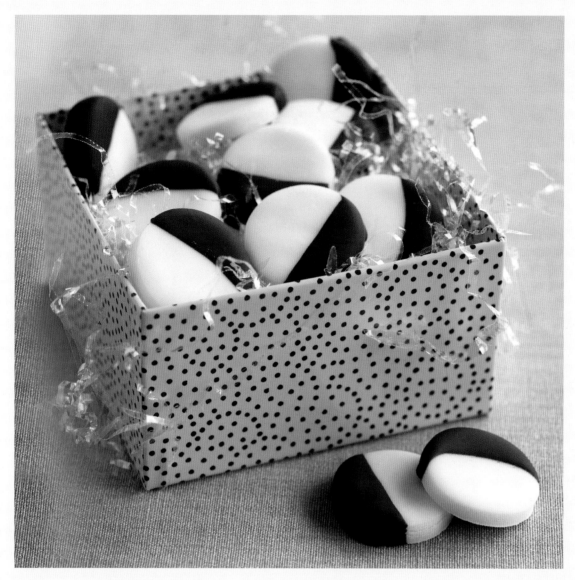

◀ If giving the peppermint creams as a gift, use some clean cellophane wrap inside a box to keep them from breaking up.

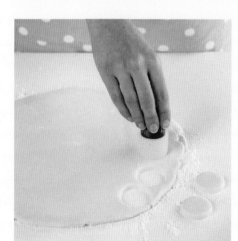

4 Roll out the mix until it is about ½in (5mm) thick. Use the cutter to cut out discs from the mix and put on the baking paper to dry.

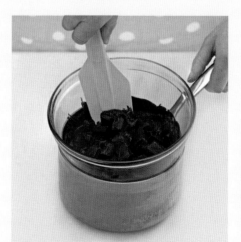

5 Break the chocolate into the heatproof bowl. Bring a pan of water to simmering, place the bowl over it, and allow the chocolate to melt.

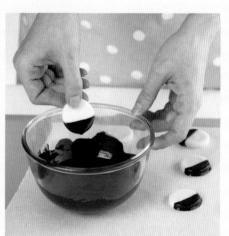

6 Take the bowl off the heat. Dip each sugar disc so that it is half-covered in chocolate and place it on the parchment paper to harden.

Useful resources

AARP Resources

AARP.org/health/brain-health/

There is a lot of advice about brain health out there. That's why the Global Council on Brain Health and Staying Sharp are cuttng through the noise and bringing you only those tools and information that are supported by science.

Staying Sharp

stayingsharp.org
Access to personalized science-based activities, challenges, and recipes designed to promote brain health and improve your life.

Global Council on Brain Health

GlobalCouncilOnBrainHealth.org
An independent collaborative, convened by AARP, of scientists, health professionals, scholars, and policy experts from around the world working in areas of brain health related to human cognition.

UNITED STATES

Aging Life Care Association

3275 W. Ina Road, Suite 130, Tucson, AZ 85741-2198. Tel: (520) 881 8008.
www.aginglifecare.org

Alzheimer's Association

225 N. Michigan Ave., Fl. 17, Chicago, IL 60601-7633. 24-hour helpline:
1 (800) 272 3900.
www.alz.org

Alzheimer's Foundation of America

322 Eighth Avenue, 7th Floor, New York, NY 10001.
Toll-frcc helpline: (866) 232 8484.
www.alzfdn.org

Association for Frontotemporal Degeneration (AFTD)

Radnor Station Building 2, Suite 320, 290 King of Prussia Road, Radnor, PA 19087.
Toll-free helpline: (866) 507 7222.
www.theaftd.org

Dementia Mentors

17244 HWY US, 41 Spring Hill, FL 34610.
Tel: (352) 345 6270.
www.dementiamentors.org

Dementia Society of America

PO Box 600, Doylestown, PA 18901.
1-800-DEMENTIA
www.dementiasociety.org

Lewy Body Dementia Association (LBDA)

912 Killian Hill Road S.W., Lilburn, GA 30047.
LBD Caregiver Link, tel: (800) 539 9767.
www.lbda.org

World Health Organization (WHO)

www.who.int/mental_health/neurology/dementia

CANADA

Alzheimer Society of Canada
20 Eglinton Ave. W., 16th Floor, Toronto, ON M4R 1K8
1-800-616-8816
alzheimer.ca

Alzheimer's Association
alz.org/ca

Lewy Body Dementia
www.lewybodydementia.ca

Memory Loss Foundation
memorylossfoundation.ca

Mount Sinai Hospital (Toronto) Dementia Support Program
www.mountsinai.on.ca/care/psych/patient-programs/
geriatric-psychiatry/dementia-support/dementia-
support

Resources for Seniors—Government of Canada
www.canada.ca/seniors

Select bibliography
Dementia Fact Sheet, World Health Organization, 2017. "Exercise interventions for cognitive function in adults older than 50: A systematic review with meta-analysis," JM Northey, N Cherbuin, KL Pumpa, DJ Smee, B Rattray, *British Journal of Sports Medicine*, 2018, 52:154–160. "The global impact of dementia: An analysis of prevalence, incidence, cost and trends," *World Alzheimer Report 2015*, Prof. M Prince, Prof. A Wimo, Dr M Guerchet, G-C Ali, Dr Yu-Tzu Wu, Dr M Prina, Alzheimer's Disease International, 2015. "Is your housing dementia friendly? EHE Environmental Assessment Tool," The King's Fund, UK, 2014. "Living with dementia and connecting with nature – looking back and stepping forwards," Neil Mapes, Dementia Adventure, 2011. "Sound-making actions lead to immediate plastic changes of neuromagnetic evoked responses and induced ß-Band oscillations during perception," B Ross, M Barat, T Fujioka, *Journal of Neuroscience*, 2017, 37 (24) 5948-5959. Survey results on shopping, Alzheimer's Society, UK, https://www.alzheimers.org.uk/download/downloads/id/3064/dementia_friendly_retail_guide.pdf.

Index

Acknowledgments

The publisher would like to thank Mary Slater for her help and expertise with the knitting project; Dave King for additional photography; Emily Kimball of Penguin Random House and Tom Miller of the Carol Mann Agency for their tireless contract work; Jodi Lipson and Laurie Edwards of AARP for editorial input and guidance; and Karyn Gerhard for helping put it all together.

Author's acknowledgments
My heartfelt thanks go to all of you who have helped me along the way with writing this book. To my husband Dan and gorgeous girls, Amélie and Esmé, for all their support and patience. To Dad, and Mum, who was with me every step of the way, and my friends Hazel, Karyn, Karen, and Gwen, who kept me going during the tough times. To my editor, Annelise, who held my hand, and all the team at my publisher Dorling Kindersley. Thank you for believing in me. Thank you to all the people living with dementia and their carers, including members of the DEEP network and the health and social care professionals who provided such valuable feedback. I couldn't have done it without you.

The publisher would like to thank the following for their kind permission to reproduce their photographs:

(Key: a-above; b-below/bottom; c-center; f-far; l-left; r-right; t-top)

5 Getty Images: Frank Gaglione (tc). 6 Getty Images: Amit Somvanshi (bl). iStockphoto.com: Kali9 (br). 7 Getty Images: Don Mason (br); Klaus Tiedge (bl); Ariel Skelley (cb). 10 123RF.com: 3ddock (cb); Pixelrobot (fclb); Maxim Kazmin (crb, fcrb). 11 Dorling Kindersley: NASA (cla). Getty Images: Popperfoto (tc); Voisin (cr); Tetra Images (cb, clb). 13 Science Photo Library: Alfred Pasieka (crb). 14 Dreamstime.com: Aleksey Boldin (cr). 15 Getty Images: Ariel Skelley (b). 16 Dreamstime.com: Ljupco (cl). iStockphoto.com: Kali9 (br). 17 Getty Images: Rana Faure / Corbis / VCG (t). 18 Alamy Stock Photo: Sean Prior (clb). Dreamstime.com: Denis Fefilov (cra). Getty Images: Media for Medical (crb). 19 123RF.com: Voravan Phalasin (r). Alamy Stock Photo: Image Source Plus (bl). 20 iStockphoto.com: FredFroese (bl). 21 Alamy Stock Photo: Image Source (cr). 22 Getty Images: Image Source (br). 23 Getty Images: Cultura RM Exclusive / yellowdog (br); Steve Mason (tr). 26 123RF.com: Wavebreak Media Ltd (bc). Depositphotos Inc: Gvictoria (ca). Getty Images: Hero Images (crb); David Sacks (cb). 27 iStockphoto.com: Ferrantraite. 28 Depositphotos Inc: Monkeybusiness (bl). Dreamstime.com: Dennis Van De Water / Dennisvdwater (cb). iStockphoto.com: MarioGuti (br). 29 Depositphotos Inc: Nullplus. 30 Alamy Stock Photo: Doc-Stock (cb). Dreamstime.com: Tombaky (bl). Getty Images: Jupiterimages (br); Tetra Images (ca). 31 Getty Images: Steve Mason. 32 Getty Images: Lisa Blumenfeld / Staff (tr); George Tiedemann (bl); Marcus Brandt / Staff (br). 33 Getty Images: David Cannon (br); Universal (tl); Rolls Press / Popperfoto (tr); Bob Martin / Staff (bl). 34 Dreamstime.com: Julián Rovagnati / Erdosain (ca). Getty Images: Peter Muller (bl). iStockphoto.com: Csondy (br); Photoevent (bc). 35 Getty Images: Jetta Productions (bc); SelectStock (t); Rolfo (bl). 36 Depositphotos Inc: Goodluz (br). Dreamstime.com: Kanjanee Chaisin (cb). iStockphoto.com: Gilaxia (clb). 37 Getty Images: Jose Luis Pelaez Inc. 40 Alamy Stock Photo: Jozef Polc (cb). Getty Images: Rosmarie Wirz (crb). iStockphoto.com: Adamkaz (br). 41 Dreamstime.com: Bennymarty. 42 Getty Images: Thinkstock (bc). 43 Getty Images: Echo. 44 Getty Images: Aluma Images (bc); Michael Kirby / EyeEm (crb); Kathy Collins (br). 45 Getty Images: Guido Cozzi / Atlantide Phototravel. 46 Getty Images: Marc Romanelli (br). 47 Getty Images: Andrew Peacock

(bl). 48 Getty Images: Cultura RM Exclusive / yellowdog (crb). iStockphoto.com: AzmanJaka (cb). 49 Getty Images: ML Harris. 50 123RF.com: Dmitriy Shironosov (br). Getty Images: Klaus Vedfelt (c). 51 123RF.com: Auremar (br). Alamy Stock Photo: LJSphotography (bl). Getty Images: Image Source (t); Betsie Van Der Meer (bc). 52 Getty Images: Horst P. Horst (r). 53 Getty Images: Nick Dolding (bl); Popperfoto (tl); Gems (tr); Paul Harris (br). 54 Dreamstime.com: Monkey Business Images (crb). Getty Images: Daqiao Photography (crb); Richard Maschmeyer (cb); David Sacks (br). 55 Getty Images: Billy Stock / Robertharding. 56 iStockphoto.com: Malerapaso (t); Mladn61 (bl). 57 Getty Images: 709122029 (bl). iStockphoto.com: Venakr (t); skodonnell (bc). 59 iStockphoto.com: AleksandarNakic. 61 Dorling Kindersley: Matthew Ward (b). 62 123RF.com: Weerapat Wattanapichayakul (clb). Getty Images: Kim Sayer (br). 63 Getty Images: Ron Sutherland. 64 Getty Images: Mark Turner (bc). 65 Alamy Stock Photo: Clare Gainey (bc); Dave Zubraski (t). Dorling Kindersley: Mark Winwood / RHS Wisley (bl). 66 Dreamstime.com: Tracy Decourcy (ca). 67 Dreamstime.com: Aliaksandr Mazurkevich. 70 iStockphoto.com: KenCanning. 71 Dreamstime.com: Romano Petešić / Shandor (ca). Getty Images: Brigitte Sporrer (bc). iStockphoto.com: Buburuzaproductions (crb). 72 Alamy Stock Photo: Deborah Vernon (bc). Dorling Kindersley: Fotolia: Thomas Dobner / Dual Aspect (ca). Getty Images: Andrew Howe (clb). iStockphoto.com: Cisilya (crb). 74 Getty Images: Itsabreeze Photography (tc). 82 iStockphoto.com: Eclipse_Images. 83 iStockphoto.com: Catscandotcom (clb). 84 Getty Images: Daniel Ingold (bc). iStockphoto.com: Catscandotcom (bl); Ugurhan (br). 85 Depositphotos Inc: Syda_Productions (br). Getty Images: Hill Street Studios (t). iStockphoto.com: Shironosov (bc). 86 Alamy Stock Photo: Juice Images (cb). Dreamstime.com: Ovydyborets (crb/Background). iStockphoto.com: Leremy (crb). 88 iStockphoto.com: Whitemay (br). 89 Getty Images: Laurie Rubin (bc). iStockphoto.com: JohnGollop (bl); Wragg (t). 90 Getty Images: H. Armstrong Roberts / ClassicStock (clb); Jeff Greenberg (fclb); Education Images (fcrb); David Redfern / Staff (crb). 91 iStockphoto.com: Fstop123. 92 Dreamstime.com: Ian Poole / Ianpoole (c). 93 Dreamstime.com: Manaemedia / iPhone® is a trademark of Apple Inc., registered in the U.S. and other countries. (br). 94 Getty Images: Ryan Etter (bc); Chris Tobin (br). iStockphoto.com: Antonio D'Albore (ca). 95 Dorling Kindersley: Ruth Jenkinson / Ruth Jenkinson Photography (t). Getty Images: Images by Fabio (bl). iStockphoto.com: Leezsnow (bc). 96 Depositphotos Inc: Isantilli (bl). Dreamstime.com: Goir (bc). iStockphoto.com: Didecs (br). 98 Alamy Stock Photo: Granger Historical Picture Archive (br); Robertharding (clb). Getty Images: Bettmann (cb). 99 Getty Images: Movie Poster Image Art. 101 Getty Images: ATU Images (br). 104 Getty Images: Merten Snijders (bc); Terry Vine (clb). Rex by Shutterstock: Hans Von Nolde / AP (br). 105 Alamy Stock Photo: Everett Collection Inc. 106 Getty Images: Richard E. Aaron (clb); Digital Vision (cb); Jack Vartoogian (bc); Paul Popper / Popperfoto (br). 107 Dreamstime.com: Volodymyr Shevchuk. 108-109 Alamy Stock Photo: World History Archive. 110-111 iStockphoto.com: RG-vc (b). 111 Getty Images: Nick Dolding (tr). iStockphoto.com: FangXiaNuo (t). 112 Getty Images: BJI / Blue Jean Images (br); Blend Images - KidStock (clb); Jose Luis Pelaez Inc (cb). 113 Getty Images: Sunset Boulevard. 114 Alamy Stock Photo: Pictorial Press Ltd (crb). Getty Images: Constance Bannister Corp (bc); Lambert (fclb). iStockphoto.com: Cclickclick (t). 115 Dreamstime.com: Alextan8 (l). Getty Images: Peter Dazeley (bl). iStockphoto.com: Allanswart (cb); FireAtDusk (cra). 116 Getty Images: Imagenavi (ca); Mary Smyth (b). iStockphoto.com: J-Elgaard (cb); Sutteerug (bc). 117 Getty

Images: Sappington Todd. 120 Alamy Stock Photo: Zoonar GmbH (c). iStockphoto.com: Ermingut (ca). 122 Dreamstime.com: Epicstock (bl); Melinda Nagy / Melis (br). Getty Images: Thomas Imo (clb). iStockphoto.com: PamelaJoeMcFarlane (bc). 124 Getty Images: Michelle Arnold / EyeEm (fclb); Dimitri Otis (crb). 125 Getty Images: Frank Gaglione. 126 123RF.com: Siraphol (bc). 127 Depositphotos Inc: Ssuaphoto. 128 Alamy Stock Photo: Juice Images (crb). Getty Images: Stockbyte (ca). iStockphoto.com: Joas (cb). 129 iStockphoto.com: Nano. 130 Dreamstime.com: Yuliya Ermakova / Julialine (fclb). Getty Images: Michael Dunning (br). iStockphoto.com: AMR Image (cb); Bhofack2 (bc). 131 Dorling Kindersley: Dave King / The Science Museum, London (clb). Dreamstime.com: Assoonas (c). 132-133 Dorling Kindersley: NASA. 134 Depositphotos Inc: Ajafoto (ca). Getty Images: Peter Dazeley (bc). iStockphoto.com: Franckreporter (crb); Sorastock (cb). 135 iStockphoto.com: Bauhaus1000. 136 123RF.com: Stylephotographs (bl). Dreamstime.com: Valeriia Samarkina (bl). Getty Images: Lee Dawkins / EyeEm (bc). 137 Alamy Stock Photo: Nutmeg Photos, LLC (t). Dorling Kindersley: E.J. Peiker (cb). Dreamstime.com: Nomadimages (bc/Multiple Images); Rhallam (bc). Getty Images: Vince Talotta (br). iStockphoto.com: Hillwoman2 (bl). 138 Alamy Stock Photo: PhotoStock-Israel (ca). Dreamstime.com: Adam88x (br). 139 iStockphoto.com: Lisegagne. 140 Dorling Kindersley: Barnabas Kindersley (cra). Dreamstime.com: Yuri Yavnik / Yoriy (crb). 140-141 Dreamstime.com: Pixattitude. 141 Dreamstime.com: Sorin Colac (clb); Jarnogz (cra). 142 Getty Images: Dimitri Otis (crb); Tooga (ca). 143 123RF.com: Andriy Popov (bc). iStockphoto.com: Diego_cervo (t); Submethod (bl); Lebazele (br). 144 123RF.com: Robinsphoto (bl). Alamy Stock Photo: Wavebreak Media (br). 145 Alamy Stock Photo: Asia Images Group Pte Ltd. 146 Dorling Kindersley: Matthew Ward / Owned by Ian Shanks of Northamptonshire (cb). Dreamstime.com: Neophuket (br). 152 Alamy Stock Photo: Wavebreak Media ltd (bc); Edward Westmacott / Stockimo (br). 153 Alamy Stock Photo: Lev Dolgachov (br); Zoonar GmbH (bl). iStockphoto.com: ChristiLaLiberte (t). 158 Dreamstime.com: Hywit Dimyadi / Photosoup (tr). 159 Dreamstime.com: Hywit Dimyadi / Photosoup (tl, tc, tr); Torsakarin (tr/Background). 161 iStockphoto.com: Davincidig (br); Petekarici (bl); Wavebreakmedia (bc). 164-165 Bridgeman Images: A Sunday on La Grande Jatte, 1884-86 (oil on canvas), Seurat, Georges Pierre (1859-91) / The Art Institute of Chicago, IL, USA / Helen Birch Bartlett Memorial Collection. 167 iStockphoto.com: Bloodlinewolf. 174 Dorling Kindersley: Gary Ombler / J J Guitars (bl). Getty Images: Enrique Ramos López / EyeEm (crb). 175 iStockphoto.com: Zoran Zeremski. 176 Getty Images: MOAimage (br). 180-181 Getty Images: Ullstein bild. 183 Dreamstime.com: 7191052k (bc). Getty Images: Ashley Cooper (br); Rae Russel (bl). 184 Getty Images: Rosemary Calvert (ca); (C) Maite Pons (cb). iStockphoto.com: DragonImages (bc). 185 iStockphoto.com: Mkovalevskaya. 188 Getty Images: Diane Macdonald (b). 189 Getty Images: Westend61. 192 Alamy Stock Photo: Studiomode (br). 193 iStockphoto.com: Clark_Fang. 194 iStockphoto.com: Ramajoo (cb). 199 Dreamstime.com: Fuzzbass (cra). 200 Getty Images: Eddy Zecchinon / EyeEm (br). iStockphoto.com: Bonchan (bc). 201 Getty Images: Cultura RM Exclusive / Flynn Larsen (br); Maria Fuchs (c); Juliette Wade (br). 204 iStockphoto.com: DNY59 (ca). 205 Getty Images: Roy Mehta. 208 Getty Images: Doerte Siebke / EyeEm (br). 209 Getty Images: Jose Luis Pelaez Inc. 210 Getty Images: Diana Miller (br). 211 Getty Images: James Baigrie.

All other images © Dorling Kindersley
For further information see:
www.dkimages.com